"This book provides a fascinating and illuminating exploration of the vital hidden assumptions in psychological theory, research, and practice. Slife, O'Grady, and Kosits have assembled an accessible, concise, must-read text for every psychologist and student of psychology. They wisely show us how our preconceptions guide our professional work without suggesting that we can purify that work of our grounded humanity."
—**Blaine J. Fowers**, *Professor of Counseling Psychology,*
University of Miami, USA

"Those of us who turn to the science of psychology for empirically-based answers concerning how to be a good person and lead a good life inevitably will be disappointed. The chapters in this splendid book explain why."
—**Jack Martin**, *Burnaby Mountain Endowed Professor*
of Psychology, Simon Fraser University, Canada

"A duty of theoretical and philosophical psychology is to expand the boundaries of the discipline, profession, and our horizons. This book impressively accomplishes this task by focusing on the relevance of unquestioned worldviews in theory and practice. Karl Jaspers would have been intrigued."
—**Thomas Teo**, *Professor in the History of Theory*
of Psychology Program, York University, Canada

The Hidden Worldviews of Psychology's Theory, Research, and Practice

By revealing underlying assumptions that influence the field of psychology, *The Hidden Worldviews of Psychology's Theory, Research, and Practice* challenges psychologists to reconsider the origins of ideas they may take as psychological truths. Worldviews, or the systems of assumptions that provide a framework for psychological thinking, have great influence on psychological theory, research, and practice. This book attempts to correct assumptions by describing the worldviews that have shaped psychological theory, practice, and research and demonstrating how taking worldviews into account can greatly advance psychology as a whole.

Brent D. Slife is Professor of Psychology, Brigham Young University, USA and the present Editor-in-Chief of the APA *Journal of Theoretical and Philosophical Psychology*. He has authored over 200 articles and 10 books, and continues his psychotherapy practice of over 30 years.

Kari A. O'Grady is Associate Professor of Psychology and Pastoral Counseling, Loyola University Maryland, USA. She is the director for the Center for Trauma Studies and Resilience Leadership.

Russell D. Kosits is Associate Professor and Chair of Psychology, Redeemer University College, Canada.

Advances in Theoretical and Philosophical Psychology
Series Editor: Brent D. Slife
Brigham Young University

Editorial Board

The Hidden Worldviews of Psychology's Theory, Research, and Practice
Edited by Brent D. Slife, Kari A. O'Grady, and Russell D. Kosits

The Hidden Worldviews of Psychology's Theory, Research, and Practice

Edited by
Brent D. Slife, Kari A. O'Grady,
and Russell D. Kosits

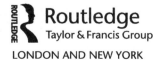

LONDON AND NEW YORK

First published 2017 by Routledge

2 Park Square, Milton Park, Abingdon, Oxfordshire OX14 4RN
52 Vanderbilt Avenue, New York, NY 10017

Routledge is an imprint of the Taylor & Francis Group, an informa business

First issued in paperback 2019

Library of Congress Cataloging-in-Publication Data
Names: Slife, Brent D., editor. | O'Grady, Kari Ann, 1969– editor. |
    Kosits, Russell D., editor.
Title: The hidden worldviews of psychology's theory, research, and
    practice / edited by Brent D. Slife, Kari A. O'Grady, and Russell D. Kosits.
Description: 1 Edition. | New York : Routledge, [2017] | Series: Advances
    in theoretical and philosophical psychology | Includes bibliographical
    references and index.
Identifiers: LCCN 2017007670 | ISBN 9781138229655 (hardback : alk.
    paper) | ISBN 9781315283975 (ebook)
Subjects: LCSH: Psychology. | Psychology—Research. | Psychology—
    Philosophy.
Classification: LCC BF121 .H493 2017 | DDC 150.1—dc23
LC record available at https://lccn.loc.gov/2017007670

ISBN: 978-1-138-22965-5 (hbk)
ISBN: 978-0-367-27115-2 (pbk)

Typeset in Times New Roman
by Apex CoVantage, LLC

To the love and light of my life, Karen.

Brent D. Slife

To my darlings Steve, Amanda, Brenna, Tommy, Daniel,
Patrick, Miles, Caleb, and my sweetheart Doug.

Kari A. O'Grady

To the memory of my father, Roger A. Kosits

Russell D. Kosits

Contents

Series Editor's Foreword

Psychologists need to face the facts. Their commitment to empiricism for answering disciplinary questions does not prevent pivotal questions from arising that cannot be evaluated empirically, hence the title of this series: *Advances in Theoretical and Philosophical Psychology*. Such questions as: What is the relation between mind and body? What is the nature of a good life? And even: Are current psychological methods adequate to truly understand the person? These questions are in some sense philosophical, to be sure, but the discipline of psychology cannot advance even its own empirical agenda without addressing questions like these in defensible ways. Indeed, it could be argued that there is no empirical evidence for the epistemology of empiricism itself!

How then does the discipline of psychology deal with such non-empirical questions? We could leave the answers exclusively to professional philosophers, but this would mean that the conceptual foundations of the discipline, including the conceptual framework of empiricism itself, is left to scholars who are *outside* the discipline. As undoubtedly helpful as philosophers are and will be, this situation would mean that the people doing the actual psychological work, psychologists themselves, are divorced from the people who formulate and re-formulate the conceptual foundations of that work. This division of labor would seem dangerous to the long-term viability of the discipline.

Instead, the founders of psychology—thinkers such as Wundt, Freud, and Spencer—recognized the importance of psychologists themselves in formulating their own foundations. These parents of psychology not only did their own theorizing, in cooperation with many others; they realized the significance of constantly re-examining these theories and philosophies, including the theories and philosophies of psychology's methods. The people most involved in the discipline's activities would thus be the ones most knowledgeable about whether and how such changes needed to be made.

This series is dedicated to this examining and re-examining of these foundations. It identifies the pivotal and problematic non-empirical issues that face the discipline and addresses these issues in the tradition of the theorists of natural science—excavating the implicit concepts and hidden assumptions of programs of research and strategies of practice to compare them to concepts and assumptions that might be better.

The present book is an important part of this project. As an exploration of worldviews, it excavates whole systems of implicit assumptions in psychology. It describes how psychologists acquire these worldviews without awareness, identifies prominent worldviews in psychological practice and research, explains the relation of these worldviews to culture and cultural studies, and offers psychologists a path toward greater disciplinary reflexivity about implicit assumptions and their worldview connections. All in all, this first volume is a wonderful way to begin our series on *Advances in Theoretical and Philosophical Psychology.*

Brent D. Slife

1 Introduction to Psychology's Worldviews

Brent D. Slife, Kari A. O'Grady, and Russell D. Kosits

Psychologists often forget that there are ideas behind their ideas. Sometimes called assumptions or presuppositions, these ideas are a hidden but influential guide or framework for how psychologists should think and what psychologists should do. This book is concerned with whole systems of these assumptions—what some would call *worldviews*.

Unfortunately, when psychologists forget about or do not acknowledge the influences of worldviews, it is tempting to think that their impact is slight or even absent. This thinking is especially tempting in psychological research where the data and investigations are frequently presented as "objective"—implying that the research is or should be relatively unbiased or free of values and assumptions. Worldviews are also rarely recognized in the formulation of psychology's many theories and practices. Personality theories, for example, are typically described as if the worldview present in the theorist's culture does not inform the personality theory formulated. And, of course, the concrete implications of these theories are often applied in the many practices of psychologists, from therapy to parenting.

Defining Worldview

Pop the word "worldview" into Google, and you will get this definition: "a particular philosophy of life or conception of the world." *Merriam-Webster's* dictionary elaborates on this understanding:

> The German word *Weltanschauung* literally means "world view"; it combines "Welt" ("world") with "Anschauung" ("view"), which ultimately derives from the Middle High German verb *schouwen* ("to look at" or "to see"). When we first adopted it from German in the mid-19th century, "weltanschauung" referred to a philosophical view or apprehension of the universe, and this sense is still the most widely used. It can also describe a more general ideology or philosophy of life.

In the field of psychology, Mark Koltko-Rivera (2004) proposed that we study worldviews as a psychological construct. His definition is helpful, and consistent with the dictionary definitions above. A worldview, he writes, is:

> a set of beliefs that includes limiting statements and assumptions regarding what exists and what does not . . ., what objects or experiences are good or bad, and what objectives, behaviors, and relationships are desirable or undesirable. A worldview defines what can be known or done in the world, and how it can be known or done. . . . Worldviews include assumptions that may be unproven, and even unprovable, but these assumptions are superordinate, in that they provide the epistemic and ontological foundations for other beliefs within a belief system.
>
> (p. 4)

In view of these definitions, we suggest that a worldview is a set of beliefs (articulated or not) on issues that are philosophical (epistemological, ethical, and ontological) in nature. We can see all three of these in Koltko-Rivera's definition. Epistemologically, worldviews define "what can be known" and "how it can be known." Ethically, they define what is "good and bad," "desirable or undesirable." Ontologically, they define "what exists and what does not," including our view of human nature. We would only add that these beliefs are not necessarily encapsulated or closed to other belief systems; worldviews are open to other worldviews, and thus can change over time.

Power of Worldviews in Psychology

Worldview beliefs also have a powerful impact or relationship to other beliefs. They are more "deeply ingressed" (Wolterstorff, 2001, p. 235) in the sense that changing them entails the revision of other beliefs. (Indeed, we may say that the more deeply ingressed a belief, the more "worldview-ish" it is). Along these lines, Koltko-Rivera says they are "superordinate," providing "foundations for other beliefs within a belief system." Worldviews often play the role of an implicit "faith" that researchers and therapists just "know," but cannot prove. (We will provide a few examples of these unproven worldview beliefs in the next section.) As such, much psychological theory, research, and practice is shaped by unexamined epistemological, ethical, and ontological worldview assumptions and values passed down through a psychologist's education and training.

It is worth noting that Koltko-Rivera's call to rigorous investigation of worldview has largely gone unheeded, which introduces a tremendous irony: We psychologists pride ourselves in our ability to explain human behavior; and yet, if worldview is a powerful shaper of human understanding, this would be a significant blind spot in our understanding of that behavior. Even more seriously, if the central contention of this volume is correct—that psychology is powerfully shaped by worldviews—then psychologists are largely ignorant of the influences on their own behavior! In other words, psychology's ignorance of worldview as a psychological topic has a concerning parallel in the tendency of psychologists to be blind to the worldview that shapes their own discipline.

Chapters 2 and 5 discuss how these "superordinate" worldview influences have been shaped by the culture, preferences, geographical locations, and values of scholarly social structures over time, with groups of scholars aligning with one description of psychology over others. The most powerful and influential scholars ultimately decided the parameters of modern psychological science. These parameters explain a large chunk of the variance of what psychologists think about themselves and those they study and serve. In fact, the power of a worldview is increased because we fail to recognize it *as* a worldview. The chapters of this book—particularly Chapters 3 and 4—flesh out the claim that psychology's theory, research, and practices are significantly shaped by worldview.

Still, the point of this book is not to call psychologists to a deeper study of worldview as a psychological construct, though this is undoubtedly a desideratum. Neither is it our goal to advocate for particular worldviews, or to show that worldviews themselves are problematic. Indeed, worldviews are inevitable. Rather, the purpose of this volume is to increase psychologists' sensitivity and accountability to the influence of the worldviews of psychology, i.e., the combination of epistemological, ethical, and ontological assumptions that shape psychological research and practice.

Dangers and Benefits of Worldviews in Research and Practice

The benefits of worldviews are that they provide structure and sense to a rapidly changing and often chaotic world. Collective worldviews, such as institutional worldviews, help define shared values and preferential approaches to complex problems. Psychologists engage each other within a shared worldview that distinguishes the profession. However, worldviews can have a dark side, as they constitute biases which can become reified prejudices. As we will soon see, the contemporary worldviews that influence modern psychology can become dangerous if we assume that psychological science is fundamentally value-free and objective, that research and therapeutic methods reveal the non-interpreted truth of the world, or that all members within a discipline walk in lockstep with their worldview beliefs. This danger is, in fact, one of the primary motivations or purposes of this book—to prevent ignorance of such hidden worldviews so as to better advance the discipline.

Dangers of Hidden Assumptions for Research

Indeed, without explicit attention to the worldview assumptions of our profession, we may be likely to engage in misaligned methodologies (i.e., allegiance to one tool of methodology that does not fit the subject matter), insensitive measurement items and interview protocols (i.e., items that capture researcher values and perspectives, rather than the experiences of the participants), and underdetermined and predictable moves in our conclusions (i.e., reification or underestimation of our worldviews). Further, we are unlikely to generate truly new findings when we remain stuck inside Kuhnian "normal" (puzzle-solving) science (Kuhn, 1970) and do not consider alternative understandings of our world.

For example, as Chapters 3 and 4 describe, many psychology researchers assume that personal subjectivity can and should be separated from objectivity and that "rigorous research" means investigations that have undergone a series of checks and balances which attempt to sterilize the data from outside influences that could distort the focus of the study. We, for instance, conduct double-blind studies to prevent the researcher's familiarity with the study from confounding the findings with undue influence from the researcher. As Chapter 4 of this volume describes, this approach to research may seem like it universally defines good research, but it is important to remember it represents a worldview assumption about the role of research methods that aligns with the worldview of some but not all researchers.

Other data collection approaches have different means for ensuring rigor—even incorporating the researcher's subjectivity *into* the study's findings—that stem from some worldviews but not others. Many approaches to qualitative methods, for example, do not attempt research rigor through the elimination or minimization of bias, primarily because they consider it impossible even to minimize biases (Packer, 2010). Rather, they seek methodological rigor by identifying their biases as well as alternative biases so that they can easily modify them in the light of data to the contrary. From this alternative logic of method, the assumption that our subjectivity can be separated from the objective aspects of the world (or conversely, the assumption that it cannot be separated) can properly be viewed as assumptions and not a fact of research investigations per se.

Again, this is not to say that either approach to method logic is flawed or unproductive. Instead, as Chapter 4 points out, it is important that we know what assumptions we are making, not to mention what methodological options we have, with both ultimately depending on the nature of our study. To expose and highlight these hidden (or ingressed) worldviews, we contrast them to other worldviews in Chapters 3 and 4. Through contrasting several of the worldview influences of two dominant worldviews in psychological science, Chapter 4 illustrates how worldviews shape even psychology's research methods themselves.

Dangers of Hidden Assumptions in Practice

Certain worldview assumptions can permeate psychotherapy in ways that are not always helpful. One seemingly innocuous practice is having clients come to our offices for treatment. The assumption is that clients have their problems *within* them—within their selves, their psyches, or their brains—and so they are considered to carry around their "personalities" or "diagnoses" from one situation to another and into our offices. The home or work situations in which the problems originate are thus assumed to be secondarily important rather than inherently defining of clients and their problems. To many psychotherapists, this belief is so familiar that it may seem axiomatic or the "way things are" in dealing with clients, but as Chapter 3 will show, it is an assumption of a prominent Western worldview—liberal individualism. Consequently, Chapter 3 also compares the characteristics of liberal individualism to the characteristics of another intriguing worldview, to allow the reader to see how the axiomatic status of received practices can be challenged.

Consider also the assumption of eliminating subjectivity that we just described in psychology's research. As Chapter 3 will outline, this "value neutrality" in research methods transfers quite nicely (or quite wrongly, depending on your worldview) to psychotherapeutic methods. Epistemology in research becomes ethics in practice. Psychotherapists, for instance, are forbidden from "imposing their values" on their clients by prominent professional ethical principles (APA, ACA). This sanction against such an "imposition" may feel "right" to many readers who have been trained in the current research worldview we have just been describing, but the contrasting worldview described in Chapter 3 not only does not accept this ethical principle but also does not think it is even possible. From this alternative worldview perspective, it is wrong, and even dangerous, to think that therapists can somehow avoid valuing their values.

Similarly, this transfer of the dualism and objectivity of the evidence-based worldview has led psychotherapists to champion "openness," as if therapists should be open to all client values (Slife, Scott, & McDonald, 2016). As Chapter 3 will describe, however, this openness may be important with some clients, but it does not account for clients whose values are clearly part of their problems. To even recognize such problems of values, therapists would require therapist value-judgments from an alternative set of values, which is forbidden in the current paradigm. Moreover, what happens when an "open-minded" therapist deals with a "closed-minded" client? As Chapter 3 explains, the research is clear: open-minded therapists attempt to make closed-minded clients more like themselves, i.e., more open-minded, even to the degree that they consider the closed-minded client abnormal (Slife, Smith, & Burchfield, 2003). Again, the point here is not that cultivating openness in clients is bad; rather, the point is that this open-minded orientation, and thus its cousins of objectivity and value-neutrality, are *themselves* worldview values, not the acceptance or elimination of all values or even the avoidance of all worldviews.

Benefits of Knowing the Assumptions Behind Our Worldviews

The aim of this volume is not to portray worldviews in and of themselves as problematic. They are unavoidable. Rather the goal is to remind readers of the need to be cognizant of the influence of their assumptions in psychology. As Chapters 5 and 6 describe, we believe it is especially important to explicitly take into account these prevailing assumptions and values so that our tendency to dismiss value systems that clash with our own will not constrain the field nor harm the consumers of psychology.

By making the worldview assumptions of modern psychology explicit, we make it possible to reconsider and reconceptualize these assumptions in ways that prompt innovative solutions to complex problems. The most profound ideas for a field are typically discovered through the juxtaposition of competing worldviews (Nemeth, 1986). Since humans appear to be naturally drawn to like-minded fellows (ideological echo chambers) and toward the path of least resistance, psychologists will likely need to make concerted efforts to intentionally expose themselves to alternative worldview perspectives. This exposure can be accomplished through various means, including interdisciplinary collaborations, working in international contexts with international partners, and fully understanding books like this one (Henrich, Heine, & Norenzayan, 2010).

Chapter 6 explains how an increased sensitivity to the values and biases inherent in the worldviews of psychology will encourage the field to be more inclusive of alternative worldviews and expand psychologist's own personal worldviews. We anticipate that such stretching will lead to more sophisticated research and theory development, increased sensitivity in assessment and treatment planning, enhanced empathy toward clients, decreased countertransference of hidden assumptions and biases, increased transparency in policy, and improved efficacy in social programs. Chapter 6 explores the benefits of this worldview plurality in greater depth.

Aims of the Book

The taken-for-granted nature of worldviews can seduce us into believing that we can conduct our research and practice from a value free, "objective" position if we just tighten up our methods, whether scientific or therapeutic. This book, by contrast, not only attempts to correct this portrayal of psychology's theory, research, and practice by describing the worldviews involved in many of these activities; it also attempts to show how taking these worldviews into account can greatly advance the work of psychologists.

The book has obviously begun with this chapter's introduction to the conception and significance of worldviews generally. Chapter 2 explains how worldviews come to operate implicitly in the thinking of psychologists through their socialization in Western graduate training. Chapters 3 and 4 more explicitly describe the characteristics and practical implications of two of the most influential worldviews in Western psychology, individualism and naturalism. The worldview of liberal individualism, with its distinctive view of human nature, pervades the taken-for-granted professional values and practices of psychotherapists (Chapter 3), while the worldview of naturalism subtly influences psychology's investigations, both their research methods and data interpretation (Chapter 4). Chapter 5 then takes up the notion of worldviews in relation to culture. It challenges the notion that worldviews are just differing views of the same world, suggesting instead that ethical research and practice requires sensitivity to the nature of the differing worlds behind worldviews, especially when working with diverse populations. For psychology to reach its full promise as a discipline, Chapter 6 describes how it will need not only to become more aware of its worldview influences but also to consider adopting the more formal stance of worldview pluralism.

References

Henrich, J., Heine, S. J., & Norenzayan, A. (2010). The weirdest people in the world? *Behavioral and Brain Sciences, 33*, 1–75. doi:10.1017/S0140525X0999152X

Kuhn, T. S. (1970). *The structure of scientific revolutions.* Chicago, IL: The University of Chicago Press.

Nemeth, C. J. (1986). Differential contributions of majority and minority influence. *Psychological Review, 93*(1), 23.

Packer, M. (2010). *The science of qualitative research.* New York, NY: Cambridge University Press.

Slife, B., Scott, L., & McDonald, A. (2016, June). The clash of liberal individualism and theism in psychotherapy: A case illustration. *Open Theology, 2*(1), 2300–6579, ISSN (Online), doi:10.1515/opth-2016-0047

Slife, B. D., Smith, A. M., & Burchfield, C. (2003). Psychotherapists as crypto-missionaries: An exemplar on the crossroads of history, theory, and philosophy. In D. B. Hill & M. J. Kral (Eds.), *About psychology: Essays at the crossroads of history, theory, and philosophy* (pp. 55–72). Albany, NY: SUNY Press.

Wolterstorff, N. (2001). *Thomas Reid and the story of epistemology.* New York: Cambridge University Press.

2 The Sociocultural Dynamics of Worldviews in Psychology and Their Challenges

Eric L. Johnson

Cultures and subcultures are large-scale communities unified by a sufficient number of significant features shared by its members to give them a common social identity, including language, customs, institutions, artifacts, ways of being (thinking, feeling, experiencing, interpreting, imagining), values, norms, rules, and beliefs, a set of which can be categorized as their worldview (WV), that undergird and shape their understanding and actions. As we have seen, WVs are "systems of assumptions" (Slife, O'Grady, & Kosits, Chapter 1, p. 1), specifically, "beliefs (articulated or not) about issues that are philosophical (epistemological, ethical, ontological) in nature" (p. 2). However, because they are *assumptions*, community members vary considerably in their awareness and understanding of them, and even for those who understand them well, they often operate implicitly. They therefore often go unarticulated and unacknowledged, particularly when they are uncontested. The vague and relatively infrequent conscious activation of WV assumptions can make understanding and dialogue between members of different WV communities difficult, ironically, especially if the topic of discussion is closely related to someone's WV assumptions. In addition, once WV assumptions are well-established within a community's epistemic system, cultural members come to interpret reality and act *on their basis* and identify with them. As a result, it is nearly impossible for well-established WV assumptions to be seriously questioned, apart from an existential crisis of some magnitude—they come to form the context of the plausible. All mature human beings hold some basic WV assumptions, whether aware of it not.

Taylor (1985) has argued that humans are socially constituted beings. That is to say, our nature is such that it is shaped by our language and socialization—by the beliefs, norms, and relationships to which we are exposed and contribute. Psychology is the study of human beings by human beings. So, psychology needs to give consideration to how (1) humans in general are constituted by their beliefs and (2) how psychologists are specifically so constituted. Since WV assumptions are comprised of and reflect the deepest and most influential human beliefs, they merit inclusion in psychological research and discourse. WVs exist as objects of psychological study in their own right, as a subcategory of cognitive phenomena operating in relation to the rest of human beliefs and other cognitive phenomena. Furthermore, the specific belief content of WVs can be examined and compared with the WVs of other communities (Koltko-Rivera, 2004; Johnson, Hill, & Cohen, 2011; Obasi, Flores, & James-Myers, 2009). However, because of their fundamental importance at the interpretive base of the human belief system—constituting what is plausible—WV assumptions should be taken into account in whatever psychological research we might suppose they would be influential on the persons being investigated, for example, in many topics within subdisciplines like cognitive psychology, cultural psychology, social psychology, personality, psychology of religion, psychopathology, and psychotherapy; yet very little research has taken them into account.

In the second place, WV assumptions are relevant to psychology insofar as they affect the psychological scientists who practice the science of psychology and guide their activities, by influencing their research, reflection, writing, and teaching. This consideration, however, requires psychologists to subject themselves, and their disciplines and disciplinary practices, to systematic critical reflection with regard to the operation of these assumptions.

Psychologists have been slow to acknowledge the role of such beliefs in their discipline. However, for over half a century, philosophers of science have recognized that such beliefs affect all the sciences. Every scientific discipline is organized around the study of a specific object of investigation and includes a disciplinary community made up of investigators, scholars, educators, and practitioners; texts that describe and explain the object and its relations to other things, and the relevant beliefs, embodied practices, and rules of discourse and practice of the disciplines; along with social institutions (e.g., university departments, research centers, and publishing houses). According to Kuhn (1977), the scientists of a discipline are guided in their work by what he called a "disciplinary matrix," a normative-belief structure, shared by most members of the disciplinary community, that includes ontological assumptions and values, a specialized vocabulary and symbolic generalizations relevant to the discipline, judgments about what needs to be studied and explained, standards for good scientific practice, and exemplars (definitive scientific models) (Bird, 2000). The disciplinary matrix of a science, therefore, includes WV assumptions that pertain to the science.

Nevertheless, because the primary focus of a discipline is on its object of inquiry, disciplinary matrices and WV beliefs are rarely consciously activated or rendered explicit in the disciplinary discourse of the members of the disciplinary community, particularly if they are largely shared and uncontested. But especially given their constitutive importance in psychology—both for understanding human beings in general and for the psychologists themselves—their being made explicit would seem to be of paramount importance. In light of their role in guiding research and its interpretation, WV and disciplinary assumptions are necessary and foundational to the scientific enterprise, so that one might suppose that regular reflection upon them and discussion about them would seem to be a duty of a mature and responsible science. The same applies to clinical theory and practice. In addition, because of the ever-present possibility that the operation of implicit assumptions might unwittingly compromise and bias research, leading to the overlooking or misinterpretation of some relevant feature of reality, the fact that they are so little acknowledged would seem to be unscientific and almost lead to the conclusion that there might be some conspiracy at work.

Worldviews as a Cultural Construct

Cultural psychology provides another perspective by which to consider the social dynamics of WVs with respect to psychology. According to cultural psychologists, the knowledge about human beings found in Western psychology is less universal than was originally recognized, because of its reliance on studies of Western samples conducted by Western psychologists who were unwittingly biased by their cultural-situatedness, using methods influenced by late modern rationalism. Many psychological phenomena (e.g., perception, memory, categorization and reasoning, intelligence, narrative, motivation, emotion, sexual desire, and psychopathology) have been found to be at least partially constituted by cultural factors (Kitayama & Cohen, 2007; see also Sundararajan, Chapter 5, this volume). Psychological universals have also been confirmed in cultural psychology, but they tend to be concepts generated at a relatively higher level of abstraction (e.g., *that* humans remember), that then allow cultural comparisons to be made. Psychological phenomena closer to the lived world (e.g., *what* humans remember) tend to be more affected by cultural differences; making direct comparisons between cultures more difficult (Triandis, 2007). Complicating matters further is the fact that communicating cultures constantly influence each other, resulting in individuals and cultures that are shaped by multiple cultural and subcultural influences (Morris, Chiu, & Liu, 2015).

So, psychological science is vastly more complicated than we thought. The psychological phenomena being investigated are differentially shaped by the cultural assumptions of the target populations, and the findings are, in turn, interpreted by researchers from within their own cultural-linguistic systems (including their WVs and disciplinary matrices), and the entire investigative and communicative enterprises are dependent on successful translation and interpretation across two or more cultural-linguistic systems, a problem particularly evident when instruments developed in one culture are used to study another.

Dealing with such complexity led cultural anthropologists to distinguish between *emic* and *etic* concepts (Goodenough, 1970; Harris, 1976), the former found in only one culture, whereas the latter are found in most, if not all, cultures. As we might expect, some cultural psychologists have concentrated on emic concepts in "local" cultures and emphasized cultural difference in their research, evident, for example, in the "indigenous psychology" movement (see www.indigenouspsych.org/index.html; Sundararajan, Chapter 5). Other cultural psychologists have focused on etic concepts in order to discern the basic psychological processes that are common to all humans, while still seeking to take into account how cultures variously influence them. Both approaches are essential to a psychology that aims at comprehensiveness. Indeed, the construct validity of etic concepts studied through cross-cultural research would generally be greater than research based on findings from a single culture. The first 100 years of modern psychology could be characterized as the search for generalizable and universal laws of the functioning of human beings, and with the recent emergence of cultural psychology, modern contemporary has moved into a phase of the documentation of greater detail and specificity.

This foray into cultural psychology was conducted to give us another way to think of the psychological differences that exist between *doxastic*[1] cultures or subcultures—communities that are united by WV beliefs—rather than by more obvious cultural differentia. As suggested above, WV communities constitute a culture/subculture distinguished by their philosophical assumptions that mostly implicitly guide their understanding and activities. Just as modern psychology studied human beings for decades from its own Western cultural perspective, overestimating uniformity and universality accordingly, its own naturalistic WV beliefs were assumed for decades, resulting in the neglect of the distinct WV perspectives of the humans being studied and of the scientists studying them. We might say that WV differences among humans constitute an important class of emic concepts that are easily overlooked by cultural outsiders and their nature and relation to other beliefs are best perceived from within the culture. Consequently, psychological research in the future will need increasingly to take into account the role of WV beliefs on human functioning on both sides of the investigation. At the same time, we should also note that "pure" WV communities are becoming harder to find, since in today's global village communication and mutual influence between them is perpetual. We turn next to a new emerging are a of philosophy, social epistemology, to consider from another perspective how WVs and social dynamics are impacting psychology.

Psychology and Social Epistemology

In the West the image of the individual scientist working alone in the laboratory making a significant independent discovery has become something of a cultural archetype, yet science is actually a product of social activity, just as much as individual activity. Let us examine some of its social features.

Epistemic or Discursive Systems

Both analytic and continental philosophers have reflected on the social dimension of knowledge. According to the analytic philosopher Alvin Goldman (2011), an epistemic system is "a social system that houses social practices, procedures, institutions, and/or patterns of interpersonal influence that affect the epistemic outcomes of its members" (p. 18). Foucault, representing the continental tradition, was especially interested in intellectual or scientific disciplines and the role that discourse and rules play in such systems. "Disciplines constitute a system of control in the production of discourse, fixing its limits through the action of an identity taking the form of a permanent reactivation of the rules" (p. 224). These rules regulate the set of discursive relations and practices of a discipline that also (give) shape (to) what is seen as an object (or a feature of an object) and prioritize features, incentivizing their investigation, while rendering others unimportant, or invisible, and in some cases, heretical.

Exclusionary Rules and Practices

Foucault (1981) also pointed out that discursive (or epistemic) systems have rules and procedures that prohibit certain topics or judgments from being expressed, by labeling such expressions "uncivilized," "false," "dogmatic," or "irrational." One of the tasks of disciplinary leaders is to implement such "exclusionary rules" in their writing, teaching, editing, and speaking. In the process, they end up regulating what counts as knowledge.

Is it possible that the implicit assumptions of the WV of naturalism have unwittingly led to exclusionary rules and practices in the epistemic/discursive systems of psychology today that have constrained their shape according to those assumptions (see O'Grady & Slife, Chapter 4)?

Science and Social Relations

There are a host of ways in which the sciences are impacted by human relationships.

Testimony

Contemporary psychologists are all aware of the contribution of reason, observation, and measurement to human knowledge. However, recent philosophers of epistemology and science have pointed out that the vast majority of knowledge that people possess—*including scientists of their fields*—is based on *testimony* (Audi, 2010; Goldberg, 2012; Lackey, 2010; Zagzebski, 2012). Apart from one's own research and personal experience and reflection, the field that scientists know and professors teach is largely derived from the testimony of others found in scientific discourse, either texts (reports/attestations of research and reflection in respected [credible and legitimate] journal articles and books, and restated in textbooks) or accessed by listening to professors, colleagues/peers, and conference speakers.

Nevertheless, testimony has been shown to be frequently unreliable (Loftus, 1979). Therefore, social epistemologists have pointed out that due consideration must be given to the trustworthiness, credibility, and expertise of informants, and what to do about disagreements between "reliable informants" (Goldman, 2011). To help community members determine trustworthy, credible, and expert informants, disciplines have established criteria, labeled "indicator properties (Craig, 1990), which include methodological expertise, knowledgeableness, "playing by the rules," and so on. Though various critical theorists have shown that the use of indicator properties cannot eliminate all bias (Fricker, 2007), the development of individual and cultural knowledge cannot do without testimony, so disciplines must do their best to determine trustworthy, credible, and expert informants.

Another question to be addressed in this volume (e.g., O'Grady & Slife, Chapter 4) is the extent to which naturalistic WV assumptions are an implicit part of the testimonial package that members of the discipline of psychology received through the course of their education and training that continues to be maintained and reinforced in ongoing discursive rules and practices.

Legitimacy

To be legitimate, according to one social psychologist, is to be "in accord with the norms, values, beliefs, practices, and procedures accepted by a group" (Zelditch, 2001, p. 33). Attaining this social perception is essential in politics and business, as well as everyday life. However, legitimacy is usually taken for granted, until called into question by other members of the group for actions that reveal a member's having flouted the group's conventions, discrediting the member and causing the member to lose his or her legitimacy. When applied to a scientific discipline, having legitimacy means being an active participant in one's guild who is held in good standing by most other members, because one's discourse and practice adhere to its standards of "good science," giving no reason for suspicion about one's legitimacy.

However, it is well known that perceptions of illegitimacy can be based on unfair and inappropriate group standards. This tendency has been well-documented with regard to race, sex, the poor, and the incarcerated, among others (Jost & Major, 2001). Again, to what extent are the assumptions of naturalism included in the legitimacy standards of contemporary human science guilds, subtly constraining the actions and discourse of their members (see O'Grady & Slife, Chapter 4)?

Democracy, Majority/Minority Relations, and Expertise

In political theory, the danger of the tyranny of the majority has long been recognized (Mill, 1859/1989). A democratic approach to science considers every member of the discipline to be, in principle, a possible legitimate informant (Kitcher, 2003). However, in the past the gate-keepers of psychology (journal editors, reviewers, publishers, heads of guilds, department chairs, and influential peers) have hindered (sometimes unintentionally, sometimes intentionally) the contributions of racial and gender minorities to the field (Fricker, 2007). In a closely related vein, Duarte, Crawford, Stern, Haidt, Jussim, and Tetlock (2015) have documented an enormous imbalance in the ratio of social psychologists who favor a liberal over a conservative political perspective. As a result, they have called for greater political diversity within social psychology, suggesting that it would help expose liberal biases that currently dominate the field, open up new areas of scientific exploration afforded by novel perspectives, and reduce the mischaracterization of underrepresented groups. Duarte et al, for example, give numerous examples of how social psychology research was biased by the assumption of a liberal progress narrative in such areas as prejudice, the environment, social authority, economics, views of the military, and so on.

It would seem very likely that the same kind of bias exists with regard to WV in psychology. If so, majority-WV members might reflect on the logic of Duarte et al., exemplified also in race and gender conflicts in the field, and consider that minority status might create a unique perspective on potential injustice largely invisible to the majority, and so they might welcome intellectual debates between members of majority- and minority-WV communities because of the opportunities they create for greater intellectual diversity. Perhaps such openness would lead to a fresh evaluation of the majority's legitimacy standards, and, as with racial and gender (and eventually political?) minorities, it might encourage self-conscious, self-critical efforts within the field of psychology to guarantee that WV minorities are not being systematically excluded from discursive space, simply because they hold a less common or unpopular WV (O'Grady & Slife, Chapter 4).

But what about the WV-minority members themselves? Trimble, Helms, and Root (2003) report a "people of color racial identity" model that categorizes six ways that individuals of a racial minority may understand themselves, including *conformity* (characterized by the incapacity to perceive adverse effects of socialization on oneself and one's group and the internalization of negative socialization messages) and *dissonance* (characterized by an ambivalent awareness of one's own self or group as minority).[2] One wonders if the same kinds of pressures might be felt by *WV* minorities that can impact their personal and social identity negatively, leading some to censor themselves and the expression of their WV beliefs, in some cases even denying or renouncing them in public contexts (conferences, journal articles), having internalized the WV norms of the majority with respect to the discipline. Nevertheless, it must be conceded that there are sometimes pragmatic and even virtuous reasons for such accommodation, for example, to stay in the dialogue and to promote dialogue, respectively.

At the same time, democratic values of the inclusion of other voices have to be balanced with other considerations, for example, the greater expertise of some members in certain areas of the discipline. In addition, public criteria are needed to evaluate WVs, so that genuinely unethical WVs (e.g., fascist or racist ideologies) are not sanctioned, though such determinations are obviously fraught with complexity.

Power/Knowledge Relations

Knowledge, according to some social theorists, is necessarily related to power, particularly in the modern, scientific West. For example, within an epistemic system like a science, having knowledge translates directly into economic power (one's salary), political power (within one's department, university, guild), personal power (freedom to pursue one's goals), social power (influence on others), and disciplinary power (impact on one's discipline). The primary challenge regarding the relation between knowledge and power is that such dynamics are often masked to those with power, perhaps especially when the expressed aim of the human activity is knowledge, that is, the unvarnished truth, as in science, education, and journalism (in contrast to politics, the military, business, and sports, where the exercise of power is more obvious). According to Foucault (1984),

> Each society has its own regime of truth, its "general politics" of the truth: that is, the types of discourse which it accepts and makes function as true; the mechanisms and instances which enable one to distinguish true and false statements, the means by which each is sanctioned; the techniques and procedures accorded value in the acquisition of truth; the status of those who are charged with saying what counts as true.
>
> (p. 73)[3]

Consequently, during the last decade of his life, Foucault began referring to "power/knowledge relations" (1979, p. 27) to underscore their necessary interrelationship. One can surely appreciate such dynamics without falling into Foucault's alleged epistemological skepticism (though Dreyfus and Rabinow [1984]), for the record, have argued that Foucault successfully avoided that self-refuting position). Indeed, most psychologists have experienced the effect of power/knowledge relations in their careers.

Is it possible that those in the WV majority in the human sciences have stifled and suppressed the voice of WV minorities by unknowingly assuming a sense of legitimacy derived from their WV and enforcing rules of discourse that prohibit reference to elements of alternative disciplinary matrices based on other WVs?

Universal vs. Local Epistemic Norms

Complicating things even further is the distinction social epistemologists have made between universal and local epistemic norms. Most moderns believe that all epistemic norms are universal; indeed, it would seem to be a defining feature of modernity. Moreover, there is abundant empirical evidence of shared epistemic norms across cultures, and some minimal set of shared epistemic norms would seem to be necessary for there to be genuine dialogue between anyone. Nevertheless, as we have seen, cultural psychology has found evidence of culture-specific epistemic norms, and there are a number of areas where epistemic norms are disputed within the West, including ethics, axiology, aesthetics, ontology, and religion. At bottom, these disputes often hinge on differences in the WV assumptions of the disputants. Consider, for example, assumptions surrounding the dialectics of determinism and human agency or brain and mind, both of which are fundamental issues in psychology and far from resolved. Universalist critics (modern or otherwise) can insist that the basis of such disputes is always a function of one or more parties having an invalid assumption. The crux of the problem, however, is that people's epistemic norms are a function of their epistemic/discursive system, and in some cases one person's universal epistemic norm is another person's local, and vice versa, making strong dialogical critique seemingly incommensurable, from a WV standpoint. Critical realism, Bahktinian dialogue, and theism disincline this author to accept such a relativistic conclusion. But more to the point, rather than continuing to ignore or bracket out WV considerations from disciplinary work, psychologists might consider questioning the current hegemony of naturalism and encourage one another to be explicit about their own WV assumptions and those of their research participants, where appropriate, in the interests of advancing their disciplines (O'Grady & Slife, Chapter 4). Were they to do so, it might help to usher in a new era of WV sensitivity and awareness and in the process enrich the field of psychology immeasurably.

The Socialization of a Human Scientist

In light of the foregoing, consideration should be given to how WV assumptions get passed on from one generation to another through the socialization processes of graduate education and becoming a member of the disciplinary guild, conveyed mostly indirectly and implicitly. To begin with, to some extent everyone in Western culture is exposed to the values of science and scientism. A more intense disciplinary socialization, however, occurs during undergraduate and especially graduate training, when future members of the profession are mentored by their professors, particularly their dissertation supervisor. During their apprenticeship, students listen to lectures, read texts, discuss topics in class, write papers and get feedback, collaborate on research, and attend conferences, learning and being shaped by the complex discourse of the discipline and its implicit assumptions, mastering its practices, and absorbing its rules, much of it, as it were, by osmosis. In addition, graduate programs are inevitably hierarchical, social institutions where subtle power relations exist that can affect one's grades, dissertation acceptance, graduation, recommendation letters, and publishing record.

Through the course of these activities, certain topics are highlighted, discussed, and investigated, while other topics are neglected, and in some cases referred to disparagingly. Whether overt and intentional or indirect and implicit, the norms of this enculturating discourse are tacitly perceived and internalized, and by such means, contemporary graduate education forms its students into a certain kind of ethical participant, one who has taken on the normative beliefs, values, attitudes, and practices of one's discipline; and comes to understand the field's sense of legitimacy, avoid exclusion, and negotiate the power structures favorably, in the process learning what is highly regarded and what is forbidden within its epistemic system, so that they too can become a reliable informant and a trusted member of the intellectual majority.

Because WV assumptions are, for the most part, implicitly embedded in one's disciplinary matrix, they are communicated and absorbed mostly indirectly during graduate training. Nevertheless, they end up becoming the largely implicit plausibility structures of one's professional thought and practice. Consequently, scientists later, with a few exceptions, rarely give thought to their WV assumptions. Usually, only when the discourse rules and assumptions of one's discipline are violated or contested by someone (as is being done in this book), for example, by acknowledging the possibility of different WV assumptions than those that dominate the discipline and so raising foundational questions about legitimacy, do they get activated. By contrast, WV minority scientists are far more likely to have their basic beliefs activated regularly. As a result, WV issues will usually be more salient to them, and they will likely reflect more on them than will majority WV scientists.

WV Bias in Psychological Science?

As we have seen, implicit assumptions are necessary to make possible all complex human thought and practice. At the same time, as their basis, they cannot be proven to be true in the same way that an algebraic axiom or even an empirical pattern can. They are, rather, *taken* to be true—in effect believed, accepted, consented to—and once firmly assumed, they usually operate without conscious awareness, unless activated. Even more insidious is the possibility that WV assumptions are embedded in the empirical methods used in the field, which are nonetheless commonly believed by scientists to be WV-neutral and the very basis of objectivity.

In part, to guarantee positive knowledge, modern psychology from its founding accepted methodological naturalism (James, 1890, pp. 183–185) and early on embraced positivism (Danziger, 1979; Watson, 1913), both of which required the suppression of all WVs that were incompatible with their respective assumptions. Admittedly, this move did guarantee greater unity and consensus in the field than would have otherwise occurred. However, it must be asked: what was the cost to psychology of this commitment? Though appearing neutral, methodological naturalism and positivism restrict what counts as scientific knowledge, so they placed severe limits on what was considered legitimate in psychology for most of the 20th century by excluding much of the complexity and richness of human life, and also by its prejudice against WV-minority scientists and subjects. Perhaps the most obvious example is the exclusion of moral and ethical phenomena, which were largely absent in psychology until the emergence of positive psychology around the turn of this century. One might suppose that a human science that purports to describe the psychological dynamics of all human beings should not use methods that exclude *a priori* many aspects of the psychological dynamics of communities whose members hold different WVs. The best solution might be the field's legitimation of multiple research methods responsibly used by investigators from different WV communities delivering relatively diverse bodies of psychological knowledge (O'Grady & Slife, Chapter 4; Kosits, Chapter 6).

To provide just one illustration of this point, let us consider the construct of the self. According to a notable modern researcher, the self is defined as "how one consciously reflects upon and evaluates one's characteristics in a manner that he/she can verbalize" (Harter, 2012, p. 22). In keeping with the emphasis of much American psychology the focus is directed to individual differences in self-representations—distinctive features of the self that emerge through social interactions, individual activity, and increasing cognitive development, unfolding in modern American adults into as many as 20 domain-specific areas of self-understanding and evaluation, including intelligence, job competence, physical appearance, sociability, morality, and nurturance, among others. By contrast, consider the Buddhist concept of "no-self." Buddhists believe that humans have no independent being or essence, but are simply a collection of psychological processes, including perceptions, feelings, impulses, and consciousness. The *I* is simply a convenient label for the impermanent, ever-changing collection of an individual's experiences, but according to Buddhism, humans tragically reify this label. "The ultimate goal in Buddhism is to realize that the true nature of self is Anatman, no-self" (Ando, 2009, p. 11). The goal of human development, according to Buddhism, is "enlightenment" through the realization that one is absolutely interconnected to the entire universe and actually exists in fundamental unity of being with everything else, which results in the dissolution of the sense of the I or the Self (Engler, 2009). Or, consider a Christian approach to the self is based on a worshipful, dependent, and receptive relationship with God and the Christian's "union with Christ," by which the self-representation of Christians is fundamentally reconfigured by a loving speech-act of God (Campbell, 2012; Horton, 2011). The Christian self is essentially religious and relational, transcendently positive, but unknowable apart from faith in Christ and Christian revelation.[4]

Modern psychologists might object that Buddhist and Christian approaches to the self are importing metaphysical assumptions into their conceptions, but that is just the point. Self-representations are as psychological a construct as one can find, yet they are necessarily socially and culturally conditioned, and the metaphysical assumptions of a culture are part of its WV, including the lack of such assumptions. Modern psychologists have been socialized into what Taylor (2007) calls an "immanent" or "secular" "frame" (Chapter 15), an unconscious "picture" of reality which operates as a "background to our thinking, within whose terms it is carried on, but which is often largely unformulated, and to which we can frequently, just for this reason, imagine no alternative" (p. 549). Having absorbed this picture implicitly, it continues tacitly to shape their norms, values, beliefs, and understanding of good science, and attitudes regarding validity, soundness, and legitimacy within psychology, corresponding to the WV assumptions by which they have been largely unconsciously socialized. As a result, most contemporary psychologists have been constrained implicitly from understanding human beings in ways that transcend the limits of the minimalist and very conservative positivist epistemology and naturalistic WV to which they, at least implicitly, subscribe.

Toward a More Comprehensive Psychological Science

If it is true that humans are constituted by their beliefs, then it makes good sense for psychologists to include an assessment of the WV beliefs of research participants in studies where WV beliefs would be hypothesized to be relevant (like self-representation research). A more radical proposal, however, would be for contemporary psychology to disavow the modern ideal of a universal science of human beings "uncontaminated by WV beliefs," reject the hegemony enjoyed by the naturalistic WV, and reconceive of itself as a necessarily pluralistic science of human beings that must take into account the constituting effects of different doxastic communities and their distinctive WV beliefs (Kosits, Chapter 6). This would not affect all areas of psychology equally, but it would result in a family of approaches in those areas of psychology where WVs make a noticeable difference in the experience, functioning, and activities of human beings. One avenue for such exploration is the ideological surround research model of P. J. Watson (2011; Johnson & Watson, 2012), which includes a number of quantitative procedures for assessing the influence of WV assumptions in research programs.

Were this proposal to be accepted, it would require that graduate education and training promote greater awareness of disciplinary assumptions and include some exposure to the major WV communities there are in the world, and that opportunities be given to students to reflect on and articulate, in writing and with some sophistication, their own WV, encouraging them to consider how it might bias their understanding of human beings. Furthermore, disciplinary discourse rules would have to be renegotiated, so that psychologists are encouraged to be more explicit about their own WV assumptions, stating them up front in early sections of texts, just as best practices in many fields now require persons to acknowledge possible conflicts of interest (for example, before entering into contracts of various kinds), and depending on the topic of investigation, requiring some record of the WV assumptions of the subjects in psychological studies.

The result would be the creation of a kind of discourse space within the discipline of psychology that would be more likely to encourage all members of the field to contribute to the science according to their own WV standpoint, including members of WV-minority communities, and this would be nothing short of a scientific revolution.

Notes

1 *Doxa* means "belief" in Greek.
2 We might mention the opposite reaction to minority status that Trimble et al. (2003) report: *Immersion*—psychological and physical withdrawal into one's own group, its idealization, and the denigration of the majority culture, which can be found among fundamentalists.
3   "There is a battle 'for the truth,' or at least 'around truth'—it being understood once again that by truth I do not mean 'the ensemble of truths which to be discovered and accepted,' but rather 'the ensemble of rules according to which the true and the false are separated and specific effects of power attached to the true, it being understood also that it's a matter not of a battle 'on behalf' of the truth, but of a battle about the status of truth and the economic and political role it plays. It is necessary to think of the political problems of intellectuals not in terms of 'science' and 'ideology,' but in terms of 'truth' and 'power'"
(Foucault, 1984, p. 74).

4 Contrasting these three views of the self does not mean they are incommensurable. On the contrary, the theistic orientation of the Christian self is compatible in principle with the domain-specific features of self-representation according to Harter. The Buddhist concept of no-self is more difficult to synthesize with the other two approaches, but analogies have been explored.

References

Ando, O. (2009). Psychotherapy and Buddhism: A psychological consideration of key points of contact. In E. Mathers, M. E. Miller, & O. Ando (Eds.), *Self and no-self: Continuing the dialogue between Buddhism and psychotherapy* (pp. 8–18). London: Routledge.
Audi, R. (2010). *Epistemology: A contemporary introduction to the theory of knowledge* (3rd ed.). New York: Routledge.
Bird, A. (2000). *Thomas Kuhn*. Princeton, NJ: Princeton University Press.
Campbell, C. R. (2012). *Paul and union with Christ: An exegetical and theological study*. Grand Rapids, MI: Zondervan.
Craig, E. (1990). *Knowledge and the state of nature*. Oxford: Oxford University Press.

Danziger, K. (1979). The positivist repudiation of Wundt. *Journal of the History of the Behavioral Sciences, 15*, 205–230.

Dreyfus, H. L., & Rabinow, P. (1984). *Michel Foucault: Beyond structuralism and hermeneutics* (2nd ed.). Chicago, IL: The University of Chicago Press.

Duarte, J. L., Crawford, J. T., Stern, Ch., Haidt, J., Jussim, L., & Tetlock, P. E. (2015). Political diversity will improve social psychological science. *Behavioral and Brain Sciences, 38*, 1–58. doi:10.1017/S0140525X14000430,e130

Engler, B. (2009). *Personality theories: An introduction* (8th ed.). Boston: Houghton Mifflin Harcourt.

Foucault, M. (1979). *Discipline and punish: The birth of the prison* (A. Sheridan, Trans.). New York: Random House.

Foucault, M. (1981). The order of discourse. In R. Young (Ed.), *Untying the text: A poststructuralist reader* (pp. 48–78). London: RKP.

Foucault, M. (1984). Truth and power. In P. Rabinow (Ed.), *The Foucault reader* (pp. 51–75). New York: Pantheon.

Fricker, M. (2007). *Epistemic injustice: Power and the ethics of knowing.* New York: Oxford University Press.

Goldberg, S. C. (2012). *Relying on others: An essay in epistemology.* New York: Oxford University Press.

Goldman, A. I. (2011). A guide to social epistemology. In A. I. Goldman & D. Whitcomb (Eds.), *Social epistemology: Essential readings.* New York: Oxford University Press.

Goodenough, W. H. (1970). *Description and comparison in cultural anthropology.* Chicago, IL: Aldine.

Harris, M. (1976). History and significance of the emic/etic distinction. *Annual Review of Anthropology, 5*, 320–350.

Harter, S. (2012). *The construction of the self* (2nd ed.). New York: Guilford.

Horton, M. S. (2011). *The Christian faith: A systematic theology for pilgrims on the way.* Grand Rapids, MI: Zondervan.

James, W. (1890). *Principles of psychology.* New York: Henry Holt & Co.

Johnson, E. L., & Watson, P. J. (2012). Worldview communities and the science of psychology. In R. L. Piedmont & A. Village (Eds.), *Research in the social scientific study of religion: Vol. 23* (pp. 269–284). Leiden and Boston: Brill.

Johnson, K. A., Hill, E. D., & Cohen, A. B. (2011). Integrating the study of culture and religion: Toward a psychology of worldview. *Social and Personality Psychology Compass, 5*(3), 137–152. doi:10.1111/j.1751-9004.2010.00339x

Jost, J. T., & Major, B. (Eds.). (2001). *The psychology of legitimacy.* New York: Cambridge University Press.

Kitayama, S., & Cohen, D. (Eds.). (2007). *Handbook of cultural psychology.* New York: Guilford.

Kitcher, P. (2003). *Science, truth, and democracy.* New York: Oxford University Press.

Koltko-Rivera, M. E. (2004). The psychology of worldviews. *Review of General Psychology, 8*(1), 3–58.

Kuhn, T. S. (1977). Second thoughts on paradigms. In *The essential tension: Selected studies in scientific tradition and change* (pp. 293–319). Chicago, IL: University of Chicago Press.

24 *Eric L. Johnson*

Lackey, J. (2010). *Learning from words: Testimony as a source of knowledge.* New York: Oxford University Press.

Loftus, E. F. (1979). *Eyewitness testimony.* Cambridge, MA: Harvard University Press.

Mill, J. S. (1989). On liberty. In *On liberty and other writings* (pp. 1–116). New York: Cambridge University Press (Original essay published 1859).

Morris, M. W., Chiu, C.-Y., & Liu, Z. (2015). Polycultural psychology. *Annual Review of Psychology, 66,* 631–659.

Obasi, E. M., Flores, L. Y., & James-Myers, L. (2009). Construction and initial validation of the worldview analysis scale (WAS). *Journal of Black Studies, 39*(6), 937–961.

Taylor, C. (1985). *Human agency and language.* Cambridge: Cambridge University Press.

Taylor, C. (2007). *A secular age.* Cambridge, MA: Harvard University Press.

Triandis, H. C. (2007). Culture and psychology: A history of the study of their relationship. In S. Kitayam & D. Cohen (Eds.), *Handbook of cultural psychology* (pp. 59–76). New York: Guilford.

Trimble, J. E., Helms, J. E., & Root, M. P. P. (2003). Social and psychological perspectives on ethnic and racial identity. In G. Bernal, J. E. Trimble, A. K. Burlew, & F. T. L. Leong (Eds.), *Handbook of racial & ethnic minority psychology* (pp. 239–275). Thousand Oaks, CA: Sage.

Watson, J. B. (1913). Psychology as the behaviorist views it. *Psychological Review, 20,* 158–177.

Watson, P. J. (2011). Whose psychology? Which rationality? Christian psychology within an ideological surround after postmodernism. *Journal of Psychology and Christianity, 30,* 306–315.

Zagzebski, L. T. (2012). *Epistemic authority: A theory of trust, authority, and autonomy in belief.* New York: Oxford University Press.

Zelditch, M., Jr. (2001). Theories of legitimacy. In J. T. Jost & B. Major (Eds.), *The psychology of legitimacy: Emerging perspectives on ideology, justice, and intergroup relations* (pp. 33–53). New York: Cambridge University Press.

3   A Prominent Worldview of Professional Psychology

Brent D. Slife, Greg Martin, and Sondra Sasser

It is difficult to evaluate the conceptual state of professional psychology these days without concluding that it is extensively fragmented. In fact, the heart of professional psychology and the focus of this chapter, psychotherapy, is exemplary of this fragmentation. There are so many diverse schools, systems, and strategies of psychotherapy that they sometimes seem too numerous to count. How is it possible, then, to think that there might be a *general* understanding of the world—a therapeutic worldview—that somehow underlies or serves as a conceptual framework for most or all of them?

As it happens, a number of astute observers of the psychotherapy movement, both historical and contemporary, have long discerned the pervasive influence of *liberal individualism* as its worldview. Philip Rieff (1966/2006) and Robert Bellah (1996) have historically chronicled this influence in our Western culture and sociology, while more recently Blaine Fowers (Fowers, Tredinnick, & Applegate, 1997; Fowers, 2005) and Frank Richardson (Richardson, Fowers, & Guignon, 1999; Richardson, 2015) have described its impact in psychology and psychotherapy. We do not have the space here to thoroughly review their collective work, nor can we link every facet of liberal individualism to the conceptual assumptions of every psychotherapy approach. However, what we can do is raise readers' consciousness about the elements of this worldview, so that they can judge for themselves how implicitly influential it is.

The problem with any such "consciousness raising" is that it is extremely difficult to gain an awareness of an implicit worldview. As many scholars have noted (Fowers, 2005; Richardson et al., 1999; Bellah, Madsen, Sullivan, Swidler, & Tipton, 1996; Rieff, 1966/2006), liberal individualism is so endemic to Western society that it is often never seen or felt—it is the metaphorical water for the fish of Western culture. How do such "fish" become aware of an all-pervasive, yet almost invisible cultural and intellectual environment? How are implicit and endemic worldviews revealed and examined?

The time-honored answer to these questions is *the dialectic*, the contrasting of one set of meanings with another (Rychlak, 1976). We first describe what the dialectic is and how it can be helpful to understanding the worldview water in which most psychotherapists are swimming. We then apply this dialectic to the many implicit characteristics of liberal individualism, contrasting them with the characteristics of another worldview, *strong relationality*. Each set of contrasting characteristics is explained and exemplified, especially in regard to some of its general implications for psychotherapy.

The Dialectic of Worldviews

The revealing of "hidden" assumptions and worldviews has always been a special problem for scholars. How does one become aware of an interpretation of the world that virtually everyone in the culture takes for granted? Indeed, such a worldview can be experienced as *the* way the world is, in which case there is no reason to identify or examine it. As mentioned, the age-old answer to this question is through *contrast*, through what the ancients and even many modern scholars have referred to as *the dialectic* (Rychlak, 1976). The dialectic has many sources and manifestations, but the main reference here is to the importance of contrast in fully understanding any meaning. Indeed, the consummate dialectician would hold that meaning is more than its similarities or its synonyms. A complete comprehension of *any* meaning requires a sense of its contrasting meanings, hence the widespread practice in dictionaries of including antonyms as well as synonyms. One cannot understand the meaning of "goodness" without some understanding of "badness." To know that she's "beautiful" is to know what she'd look like if she were "ugly."

The magic of such contrasting meanings, as thinkers across the millennia have discovered repeatedly, is that they make us aware of *implicit* meanings. As a personal example, the lead author's wife opted for "soft" contacts some years ago and only then became aware of the headache she had long experienced with "hard" contacts. In other words, she was not aware that she had even *had* such a headache until she experienced the contrasting meanings (experiences of her head) of the softer contacts. Likewise, relaxation specialists will tell you that many people are relatively unaware of how tense or anxious they are until they are comparatively relaxed.

And so it is with the worldviews that saturate our understanding. They can influence tremendously all of our practical activities, but they do so without our noticing. To really notice and understand them requires some way of contrasting them, and the greater the contrast, the greater our potential understanding. Indeed, the scholars of liberal individualism have long lamented how easily this worldview is misunderstood without adequate contrast (Fowers, Richardson, & Slife, in press). For fish to understand the water of their environment, it's not enough to describe different types of water. The fish will not properly appreciate the environment they literally breathe through their gills until they have experienced a truly stark contrast, such as being jerked from the water altogether.

Similarly, psychotherapists will not properly appreciate the liberal individualist cultural environment they have been "breathing" until they experience a truly stark contrast. We do not plan the equivalent here of jerking the reader from their individualist water, but several scholars have explored a *qualitatively* different worldview, or perhaps better put, a completely different ontology than individualism—the ontology of strong relationality (Slife, Koltko, & Prows, 2013). We use the phrase "qualitatively different" because for each important characteristic of liberal individualism, strong relationality features its own contrasting characteristic, making it very useful for highlighting the many facets of liberal individualism.

Before describing these pairs of contrasting characteristics, it is important to explain the term "strong" in strong relationality. This term is not intended to mean better or clearer than weak relationality. It is, instead, a philosophical distinction that connotes a stronger form of what many Westerners typically assume is the nature of relationships, sometimes called the weak or individualist form of relationship. This weak form assumes that all individuals are *first* self-contained identities (selves, personalities) *before* they form relationships, whereas the strong form assumes that all individuals are first and always nodes or nexuses of relationships. With either form, psychotherapists can care deeply about relationships. However, the quality of the relationship is different for each. In the weak sense, people are primordially individuals who house within themselves their essential identities and only later form relationships with other identities. In the strong relational sense, people have a shared being with their contexts at the outset. Relationships are the primordial reality, and if anything is "formed" later, it is the cultural notion of individualism *from* the relationships (culture), and not the other way round.

Contrasting Characteristics

With that clarification, we can now consider the contrasting characteristics of liberal individualism and strong relationality through a table of seven characteristics (see Table 3.1). We first attempt to explain each of these contrasts, and then try to provide practical (contrasting) examples of each worldview for psychotherapy. We title each characteristic with its individualist label (e.g., "Atomism" for the first characteristic), but we also explain how the particular

Table 3.1 Contrasting Characteristics of Two Worldviews

Features	Liberal Individualism	Strong Relationism
Atomism	Individual identity is relatively independent of context and relationships.	Individual identity is dependent on context and relationships.
Autonomy	Individuals have the power and right to govern themselves and decide their own therapy goals.	Individuals and their therapy goals are and should be informed by their moral traditions.
Happiness	Individuals should pursue the satisfaction of their own desires, including happiness and well-being.	Individuals should pursue the quality of relationships and meanings.
Instrumentalism	Individuals should use the world, including people, as resources for their own ends.	Individuals should pursue moral relationships, not use people as means to an end.
Neutrality	Therapists should strive to practice in a manner that is as free of their own values as possible.	Therapists cannot help but value their values and instead should facilitate an interchange of client/therapist values.
Freedom From	Individuals should reject unnecessary obligations as obstacles to their freedom and self-expression.	Individuals should embrace obligations and duties as a key to meaning and self-development.

individualist characteristic differs from the corresponding characteristic of strong relationality.

To avoid awkward phrasings, we will also use the terms "individualist" and "relationalist" as shorthand for a person who is currently seeing the world from or facting on a particular worldview perspective. We do not mean to preclude the possibility, as we use these terms, that real people—as opposed to the theoretically "pure" individualist or relationist—can either mix these worldviews (along with many others) or use them situationally (e.g., individualism in one context and relationality in another). Again, our space is constrained, so we refer readers to the burgeoning scholarship on liberal individualism and strong relationality as we describe these characteristics (Fowers et al., in press; Slife et al., 2013).

Characteristic 1—Atomism

The first characteristic of liberal individualism is its endorsement of philosophical atomism. Atomism, as we mean it here, is the notion that all that is primary or essential about persons (their qualities) is contained within them, whether it is their biology, their cognitions or feelings, their reinforcement histories, their egos, or their personalities. In other words, there is some kind of basic identity that is within the person and experiences the "outside" world, providing continuity across the varying situations of our lives. All the basic qualities of the individual originate from this self, with relationships forming only after the individual and even then must be incorporated within the person to be influential.

This notion is, of course, part of the "individualism" of liberal individualism. Individuals are sovereign over all things concerning their lives. Indeed, the important Western concept of universal human rights stems from this characteristic (Richardson et al., 1999). The individualist perspective is also one of the conceptual bases for the laboratory tradition in the social sciences, where the best way to study individuals is to sterilize them of their surrounding situation. In psychotherapy this characteristic accounts for why we think we can treat clients in our offices and away from the contexts of their problems. These contexts—including a client's interpersonal relationships—are viewed as secondary or incidental. Clients supposedly carry their problems around within them, including their interpersonal problems, regardless of the context. Abnormal psychology texts support this definition, presenting definitions of psychological disorders such as: "A psychological disorder [is] a psychological dysfunction within an individual associated with distress or impairment in functioning" (e.g., Barlow & Durand, 2012, p. 2).

Consider the strong relationist as a contrast. Relationists are not atomistic because they view all individuals as inextricably connected to their contexts; the very being or identity of any individual is shared with the context of which they are part. To understand or study individuals fundamentally is to understand or study them in relation to this context, including their present environment, their culture or cultures, their bodies, and their histories. Even a complete understanding of a person's brain is insufficient to understand or predict him or her (or the brain). Relational neuroscientists, in this sense, would assume something like a situated cognition, where our memories are partly dependent on our computers and phones, rather than an atomistic (self-sufficient) brain (Koole & Veenstra, 2015). The qualities of any person, from this relational perspective, originate from the persons' meaningful connections with their context, implying that those qualities can fundamentally change from one context to the next. The person you know from church may be quite different from the "same" person you know at a football game. This is not to say that there is no continuity from one situation to another. Still, the continuity burden is not carried exclusively by the internal "self" or even brain; it is at least shared by relational factors such as culture, language, and embodiment (Oyserman, Sorensen, Reber, & Chen, 2009; Smith & Semin, 2007).

The most important psychotherapy implication of a strong relational approach is that the self-contained, atomistic individual is no longer the basic unit of therapy. The person's relationships, whether interpersonal (among people) or impersonal (among other aspects of their context), are the basic units. For this reason, the quality of these relationships is more important than individualist qualities such as happiness and well-being (see next section). This relational perspective is part of the impetus for the family and group therapy movements. However, many of these movements are only partially or weakly relational because families and groups are typically conceptualized as separable from their contexts.[1] Moreover, a person's qualities can drastically change across differing contexts in a relational account, meaning that few individual traits or personalities, at least as conventionally understood, are consistent across all contexts. Even diagnostic symptoms can shift—with depressives, for example, having at least contextual "moments" in which they are not depressed. Obviously, if this is true, knowledge of these moments would be pivotal to understanding these changes, however fleeting they may seem. Too often from a relational point of view, therapists focus on the episodes associated with individualist diagnoses, and momentary changes are overlooked and not mined for their therapeutic gold.

Characteristic 2—Autonomy

Characteristic 2 refers to the "liberal" part of liberal individualism. This part of the worldview is the origin of our widespread professional values of client autonomy and empowerment. Our clients should be liberated from oppressive moral traditions and authority, and should be empowered to make their own decisions, autonomously. This characteristic, as mentioned, is connected to one of the more positive aspects of individualism, individual human rights. However, it also means the individual is ultimately king over their own lives, with the individual's community or moral tradition considered secondary if not incidental or problematic. Indeed, many therapists do not view the value of autonomy as political or ideological at all; client autonomy is a "basic need" of humanity (Ryan & Deci, 2000) and an essential component of the "good life" (Chekola, 2007; Devine, Camfield, & Gough, 2008).

From this perspective in psychotherapy, individuals should have ultimate authority over the goals of their treatment (Jennings, Sovereign, Bottorff, Mussell, & Vye, 2005; Tjeltveit, 2006). Therapists can obviously discuss these goals with their clients, but they should never obstruct the client's autonomy over the therapy's ultimate objectives. Psychotherapist Hibbert describes this autonomy to her clients in the following manner: "Therapy is designed to help you discover and achieve what you truly desire, and not what anyone else desires for you" (Tartakovsky, 2016, section, para. 2). Of course, Hibbert's warning—"not what anyone else desires for you"—does not refer just to therapists. To be truly liberated in the liberal individualist sense is to be freed from any traditions that are viewed as dogmatic and potentially obstructive to one's individual freedom. Individualists particularly target traditions such as religion in this regard because these types of belief structures are frequently seen as robbing persons of the sovereignty to make decisions over their own lives.

With strong relationality, on the other hand, a portion of the context that partially constitutes any person is their moral tradition, including cultural and religious traditions. Indeed, one of the clear lessons from the growing field of indigenous psychology is that contexts such as cultures cannot be divorced from moral traditions such as religion (Kim, Yang, & Hwang, 2006). At the very least, this lesson implies that cultural competence in psychotherapy is not possible without some competence in the religious traditions of a culture. Indeed, as we will see in Characteristic 5 below, values in general are not considered avoidable or even merely subjective in psychotherapy (Brinkman, 2015). Some values matter, regardless of the prejudices of the therapist or client. Indeed, some client problems involve their values and should thus be identified if not corrected from the relational perspective.

This perspective does not mean that dogma reigns and individuals are inevitably oppressed. The individual client should clearly have a voice in therapy decision-making, and contexts of power need to be taken into account. However, the individual is not the sole or even ultimate voice in therapy decisions, because other factors of the context, including culture, moral tradition, and therapist are vital to proper therapeutic goals. Even worldviews play a role in this regard, partly because they imply a broad set of moral goals. Individualism, for instance, values individual autonomy, while relationality questions the priority of the individual and values instead quality relationships. The notion that autonomy is a basic human or biological need, in this sense, is mistaken, because it is, rather, a reification of the cultural ideology of individualism, and thus may only apply to clients of Western culture, if it applies at all.

Characteristic 3—Happiness

If individuals are or should be autonomous—the sole or ultimate decider of their lives—then they should not only choose their own goals; those goals should concern what is best for them *as* individuals. Here, as positive psychologists have demonstrated, there seems to be considerable unanimity among most individuals in the West: they want to be happy (Locke, 2002; Seligman, 2011). There are, of course, variations on this individualist theme, such as the desire to possess well-being, to flourish, to be fulfilled, etc. Whatever the concept, however, individuals should want or need whatever ultimately benefits them. Indeed, many economic models assume that it would be irrational to do otherwise (Camerer & Fehr, 2006). Other goals, such as the goals of community, are viewed as secondary if not ultimately in the service of individual goals (see Characteristic 4). Many individualists would surely entertain a mixture of communal and individual goals, but individual goals would always and ultimately be required.

Psychotherapy and psychotherapy research are also conceptualized as if their purpose is to serve these individual goals. Often without justification or defense, therapy investigators and therapy professionals *presume* the goals of therapy are some variant of individual well-being, as if this understanding is axiomatic. Consider Szymanski (2000): "Helping individuals develop subjective self-satisfaction should be the goal in any treatment program" (p. 352). The psychotherapy sub-disciplines of psychology are themselves often defined with these understandings. For example, the counseling section of the American Psychological Association, Division 17, asserts that "the practice of Counseling Psychology encompasses a broad range of culturally-sensitive practices that help people improve their well-being" (Society of Counseling Psychology, 2016). Indeed, it is this general objective of facilitating happiness and well-being that has made client depression one of the main targets of treatment. The implicit worldview of individualism means again that no justification of these objectives are needed.

In the face of the almost axiomatic status of happiness as the good and depression as the bad, it might appear provocative that strong relationality does not make happiness (or its many variations) the main goal of people or psychotherapy. The priority is simply not the individual. The priority, instead, is quality relationships—whether marriage, friendship, or community—and quality relationships do not necessarily mean happy individuals in those relationships. The lead author, for example, has been in a good marriage of more than 40 years (Slife, 2016). While it is certainly true that the quality of this marriage has been associated with our individual happiness, it is also true that if one of us became chronically ill, neither of us would be happy, even though we could still effect a quality relationship in the midst of what would be for us suffering and sadness.

In a similar manner, the strong relationist does not automatically target depression as bad. Not only are quality relationships possible with some forms of depression; some life meanings are only reachable through suffering and sadness (Fowers et al., in press). Moreover, what is popularly viewed as "depression" (e.g., sadness, emotional pain) may validly indicate life or relationship problems, and thus should not be automatically treated until its function or meaning is discerned. Depression may, of course, indicate biochemical problems, but again the relationist does not *automatically* assume that individual emotional pain and sadness are necessarily biochemical, bad, or in need of reduction at all. In this sense, the main objective of a relational psychotherapy is less about individual pain and more about healthy relationships.

Characteristic 4—Instrumentalism

With individual objectives, such as happiness, as the primary ends of liberal individualism, virtually everything and everyone else are the means or instruments of these objectives (Richardson et al., 1999). The world becomes a "resource," to use Martin Heidegger's term (Heidegger, 1977), for our own personal use and benefit. Even "helping behavior" would have to be ultimately motivated toward some individual benefit; this ultimate motive is often viewed as a byproduct of our human nature from the individualist perspective (Marsh, 2016; Kurzban, Burton-Chellew, & West, 2015). A realtor friend of the lead author was recently asked why he so regularly attended and served at church, especially when he did not believe in God. He replied as if the answer was a no-brainer: "it is my best source of referrals!" Many business strategies are clearly instrumental in this sense (Ingerson, DeTienne, & Liljenquist, 2015).

Instrumentalism may be particularly striking in the individualist understanding of marriage: its main purpose is to make the individual spouses happy. The marriage is a means, and the individuals are the ends, implying that if the individuals are not happy, the marriage is not performing its instrumental function and divorce should be a considered. Many marital researchers, in fact, attribute the high American divorce rate to this instrumentalist attitude (e.g., Fowers, 2000; Amato, Booth, Johnson, & Rogers, 2009).

Do marriage or family therapists view marriage in this individualist manner? There is certainly anecdotal evidence of this occurring. Consider, for example, this report of a therapy case from Slife, Scott, and McDonald (2016):

> When, for instance, Mary revealed some marital strife, my supervisor was quick to question whether her marriage was serving her well-being. Was it a factor in her depression? He was very clear with me that we either get her marriage working for her happiness again, or she needs to get a new mate.

(p. 599)

There is also abundant empirical evidence that this individualist worldview is involved in the professional values of many psychotherapists (Fowers et al., 1997; Tredinnick & Fowers, 1999; Fowers et al., in press; Nelson & Slife, in press; Slife, 2015). Joe Ostenson (2010) has also concluded that virtually all the psychological measures of marital satisfaction are measures of the needs and the happiness of the individuals involved, rather than a measure of the quality of the relationship itself. Even in assessment, it seems, the individual is primary.

Strong relationists would obviously disagree; our relationships and the world are *part of* our shared being from their viewpoint. To instrumentalize the world is to instrumentalize ourselves, because the others of our lives are part of our very identities. If anything, our relationships with our friends and spouses are the ends, with individuals and their particular goals as the means. The world, certainly our friends and spouses, do not exist merely as resources to benefit us. We should seek, instead, virtuous relationships with others, as Fowers et al. (in press) contend in a recent book on virtue ethics, even if individual *un*happiness is the result.

Can these virtuous relationships be assessed *qua* relationships? Unlike individualism, a relational worldview would allow psychologists to postulate their importance and then devise ways of measuring them. These assessment measures could consist of any number of approaches, from detailed observations of marital interactions to simple qualitative interviews with an eye toward relational quality (e.g., as defined by virtue ethics) rather than mere individual happiness. Individual happiness can *ensue* from a good relationship, to be sure, but it should not be *pursued* (or expected) from the relationist perspective, because the relationship is more important. The same goes for relational business practices. As expedient as instrumentalist business practices might be in the short term, they can be problematic in the long term (Ingerson et al., 2015).

Characteristic 5—Neutrality

The "liberal" in the term liberal individualism also implies another, cherished professional value—the openness or neutrality of the therapist (Jennings et al., 2005). To be truly liberated from moral traditions and value-laden dogma, according to individualism, external authority and values, whether religious or therapeutic, should be minimized. Otherwise, this authority could contravene the individual's autonomy in making important decisions (Characteristic 2). Evidence-based practices are an extension of this thinking, because they seemingly provide a way to do therapy that is considered relatively value-free or objective.

Another approach to neutrality is to facilitate the client's values and, if anything, to operate within them. As the American Psychological Association puts it, "Grounded in dialogue, it [psychotherapy] provides a supportive environment that allows you to talk openly with someone who's objective, neutral and nonjudgmental" (2016, para. 5). Indeed, the ethics of APA and ACA are clear in their declaration that therapists should never impose their own values on their clients (American Counseling Association, 2014; American Psychological Association, 2010), leaving openness or neutrality as the only option for psychotherapists.

The strong relationist, on the other hand, contends that no such openness, neutrality, or objectivity is even possible, let alone desirable. Part of the context that co-constitutes our identities and infiltrates our cultures is our values. People—including scientists, therapists, educators—cannot help but value their values, whether verbally or nonverbally, and as such the therapy process is unavoidably an interchange of client/therapist values (Fowers, 2005). Psychotherapists have long recognized the importance of therapeutic values in theory (Rychlak, 1981), but their emphasis on therapeutic openness and neutrality, not to mention scientific objectivity, belies its recognition in their practices. For this theoretical recognition to truly be applied in practice, various moral approaches and understandings of the good life would be required in therapy training, along with an explication of the values involved in the evidence-based practice movement (Richardson et al., 1999). The issue for the relationist is not so much the truth or falseness of individualism; openness could be important for many clients. The issue is understanding ideological values such as these, so they can be evaluated for the good of the particular client and context.

In this relational sense, being open and nonjudgmental as a therapist is more a particular value than a freedom from values. One way to make this point is to investigate what supposedly open or neutral therapists do when their clients are closed-minded (or judgmental). The relevant research shows consistently that open-minded therapists typically view the close-mindedness of their clients as bad or even abnormal (Slife, Smith, & Burchfield, 2003; Tjeltveit, 1999). In fact, the research confirms that these so-called open therapists attempt to change their client's close-mindedness so that their clients are more like the therapists (Tjeltveit, 1999). Therapists, in this sense, are not open to the client's closed-mindedness at all; they are teaching their own value of openness. Paul Meehl (1959), long ago, noticed this "conversion" of clients and wondered if therapists were themselves "crypto-missionaries" (p. 257), missionaries in this case for individualism. The relationist's point is that values are always involved, and thus need to be monitored.

Characteristic 6—Freedom From

Clients should not only be liberated from the values of others, according to the individualist, they should also be freed from constraints *of any kind*, within reason. Their sovereignty over their lives means that they should "get what they want." Erich Fromm (1941) noted over a half century ago that this individualist ideology leads to a well-developed sense in the West of "freedom from" all obstacles, especially if this freedom-from does not impinge on the freedom of other individuals. Perhaps the most frequent label for these kinds of practical, everyday constraints is that of *obligation*. Obligations are regularly viewed in the West as necessary at some level but definitely negative. The best vacations are obligation-free (Cook, Burnett, Hopkins, & Loeb, 2007). Conceptions of Western retirements are frequently idealized as relatively free from constraints (Edwards & Milton, 2014; Smith & Dougherty, 2012). Indeed, this freedom is one of the reasons typically cited in gathering a large retirement nest-egg: it allows a relatively obligation-free lifestyle (Fuscaldo, 2012).

The obligations of community are considered particularly onerous. They can tie us down and prevent us from what Bellah (1996) would call *expressive individualism*, the power and duty not to conform completely to societal pressures and customs and instead express our unique selves. The work of Carl Rogers was particularly influential in incorporating this humanistic understanding into psychotherapy. For Rogers the impact of society was a primary therapeutic problem that each client needed to work through to achieve self-actualization (Rogers, 1951). Therapists should increase the individual's authentic self and decrease the individual's societal constraints. As William Doherty (1999) puts it, [therapists] "see themselves as liberation fighters, for individual fulfillment against oppressive moral codes and family structures."

The strong relationist's understanding, on the other hand, is that individuals should not be liberated from these obligations and constraints, even *if* this "freedom-from" were possible. Fromm (1941) richly portrayed the kind of personal difficulties that accompany this attempt at freedom-from, something he thought was a major source of Western problems in living (Richardson, 2005). Discussing what he called the "ambiguity of freedom," Fromm argued that virtually everyone in the West has a well-honed sense of freedom from arbitrary authority and dogmatic obstacles. Yet, we are sorely lacking a corresponding sense of "freedom to" or "freedom for" that which gives some context, direction, or deeper purpose to our increased freedom and opportunity. Many is the retiree, for example, who has realized that an obligation-free lifestyle is a relatively meaningless one (Skipper International, 2013).

Psychotherapy, from this relational worldview, cannot be about decreasing the communal and obligatory, and increasing the individual and unique. The strong relationist would not reject the aim of human authenticity per se, but authenticity itself would be reconceptualized to involve the person's surrounding context (see Guignon, 2004, for an example of such contextual authenticity). Moreover, authenticity would not be understood as something all individuals should universally strive for, because their culture would be a vital factor in what authenticity might mean and whether it is important at all. For this reason, marriage and family therapies would rarely view marital and familial obligations as a problem, even for an individual's authenticity. These obligations are part and parcel of an individual's identity, and so they must be (and already are) part of their authenticity, not separate from it. In fact, the relationist would argue that no serious relationship can occur without obligations and constraints of one sort of another.

Characteristic 7—Independence

A similar, but separable conception of the liberal individualist is the person's need for independence. This conception is similar in that it could be seen as a type of "freedom from," Characteristic 6. However, it needs to be singled out conceptually because the individualist notion of independence is not just about freedom from contextual constraints and obligations; it also concerns the types and qualities of relationships that are *acceptable* to the individualist. As mentioned at the outset, many individualists value relationships very highly. However, the way these are valued and what they consider relationships differ profoundly from the relationist. Perhaps most obviously, given the previous descriptions of this chapter, individualists value relationships because they can be used instrumentally to make us happy. This type of valuing is prominent among positive psychologists (Nelson & Slife, in press; Christopher, Richardson, & Slife, 2008). For example, one of the leaders of this movement, Martin Seligman (2011), describes in some detail how relationships, including "altruistic" ones, should be used to remit an individual's depression (Fowers et al., in press).

Another important difference between the relationist and individualist views of relationship lies in their understanding of dependence. With the individualist, independence is good and dependence is bad. Even the instrumental use of positive relationships for one's happiness has important limits from this perspective. Individuals should be cautious never to get *too* involved in a relationship, because they can become dependent and put their happiness or well-being at risk. Rejection or abandonment are rarely happy events. Dependence has also been viewed negatively in developmental models, because one of the objectives of healthy development has long been to replace the dependence of the human infant with the self-sufficiency of the adult (Fowers et al., in press). These views have led many psychotherapists to vilify dependency through conceptions like co-dependency and dependent personality disorder. As many feminists have noted, there is no "independent personality disorder" in psychology, so there must be no amount of *in*dependence that is problematic to the individualist.

The strong relationist, by contrast, champions an existential dependence—the notion that we are always and already dependent; we just trade one type of dependency for others as we mature. We should, of course, avoid irresponsible and foolish dependencies, but we will never avoid or even lessen dependency because we *are* our relationships. We still depend on the grocer, the plumber, the banker, etc. Moreover, our basic identities stem from our dependencies. One of the current authors of this chapter is a sister, cousin, girlfriend, student, etc.—all of which define who she is and what she does from this relational viewpoint. Indeed, the relationist would argue that there really is no love or intimacy *without* dependency. We are thus necessarily and existentially at risk when we truly care, with relational pain and even unhappiness a likely result. From this perspective, we should jump off the happiness bandwagon, cease our instrumentalizing of relationships, and consult our moral traditions to decide which dependencies are good and which are bad.

From the vantage of relational psychotherapy, the feminist notion of an independent personality disorder is a distinct possibility, especially in the West. If relationships are what make our lives truly meaningful, then healthy dependencies should be fostered, not avoided. Indeed, if anything, given the dominance of individualism in the West, it is likely that skills of independence have been facilitated through our development and culture, with skills of healthy dependence sorely lacking. This relative absence of dependence skills would also imply the probability of decreased interpersonal intimacy, not to mention decreased *im*personal intimacy, where the ability to "commune with nature," for example, is diminished. Needless to say, the capacity to love and be loved—perhaps the sine qua non of many relational aspirations—would also be diminished. Part of the job of these psychotherapists, then, is to facilitate these skills of dependence so that healthy, if not intimate and loving relationships can occur.

***

At this point, there is surely no doubt about the profound differences between individualism and relationality, but is individualism influential in the practical enterprise of psychotherapy? As mentioned at the outset, the answer to this question will have to be left primarily to the reader, because space constraints prevent us from explicitly connecting the seven characteristics of liberal individualism to each of the scores of therapy strategies and modalities. (See the work of Richardson (2005) and Fowers (2000) for some explorations of these relationships.)

Even so, the influence of these characteristics is surely apparent in the pervasive themes of many *informal* psychotherapeutic practices and values. These themes include: clients seen almost exclusively in therapist offices, individual well-being as a prominent therapy objective, client autonomy and empowerment as important professional values, positive relationships considered instruments of individual happiness, client values as more important than therapist values in treatment, a well-developed sense of freedom-from external authority without a comparable sense of freedom-for, and a general suspicion if not fear of interpersonal dependency.

We should clarify that we are not contending that liberal individualism is the *sole* cause of these themes, nor are we arguing that they are without exceptions in practice. Worldviews such as individualism can easily work together with other influences that will either complement and strengthen their characteristics or detract and diminish them. As an example of the former, consider how individualism's promotion of value-neutrality in therapy complements the objectivism of psychology's neopositivist philosophy of science (Brinkmann, 2015; Slife & Williams, 1995). As an example of how other factors can reduce individualism's influence, consider how the therapist's intuition of the import of relationships (e.g., "relationship heals") has sometimes diminished the usual emphasis on instrumentalism or individual happiness (e.g., divorce is not good even if it means individual unhappiness). In either case—the strengthening of individualism's influence or its relative reduction—our claim is that liberal individualism is a significant, if not vital part of these themes and often serves to justify them, especially when this influence and justification are not fully recognized or examined.

Note

1 Another distinction between individualism and strong relationality is their understanding of the parts or members of a human system. In individualism, the qualities of the system parts stem from their inherent properties—such as each person's biology or their personalities—which then interact to form the system. However, in strong relationality, the qualities of each part stem from its relationship to the other parts. The head of a stick person, for example, does not get its "headness" quality solely from its circular shape; its headness comes in part from its relationship to the rest of the figure. Similarly, my "West Texas" accent (where "accent" has three syllables) would not be noticed in West Texas, because its qualities do not stem from my inflection or enunciation but rather from its relationship with its surrounding context. In this strong relational sense, the relationship is primary, not the thing itself, even in a collection of things.

References

Amato, P. R., Booth, A., Johnson, D. R., & Rogers, S. J. (2009). *Alone together: How marriage in America is changing*. Cambridge, MA: Harvard University Press.

American Counseling Association. (2014). *ACA code of ethics*. Alexandria, VA: Author.

American Psychological Association. (2010). *Ethical principles of psychologists and code of conduct*. Retrieved on September 28, 2016, from http://apa.org/ethics/code/

American Psychological Association. (2016). *Understanding psychotherapy and how it works*. Retrieved on September 10, 2016, from www.apa.org/helpcenter/understanding-psychotherapy.aspx

Barlow, D. H., & Durand, V. M. (2012). *Abnormal psychology: An integrative approach, seventh edition*. Stanford, CT: Cengage Learning.

Bellah, R. N., Madsen, R., Sullivan, W. M., Swidler, A., & Tipton, S. M. (1996). *Habits of the heart: Individualism and commitment in American life: Updated edition with a new introduction*. Berkeley: University of California Press.

Brinkmann, S. (2015). Perils and potentials in qualitative psychology. *Integrative Psychological & Behavioral Science, 49*(2), 162–173. doi:10.1007/s12124-014-9293-z

Camerer, C. F., & Fehr, E. (2006). When does 'Economic Man' dominate social behavior? *Science, 311*(5757), 47–52. doi:10.1126/science.1110600

Chekola, M. (2007). Happiness, rationality, autonomy and the good life. *Journal of Happiness Studies, 8*(1), 51–78.

Christopher, J. C., Richardson, F. C., & Slife, B. D. (2008). Thinking through positive psychology. *Theory & Psychology, 18*(5), 555–561. doi:10.1177/0959354308093395

Cook, S. D., Burnett, T. T., Hopkins, S., & Loeb, P. (2007). *The ideal American vacation trip: An in-depth analysis of American leisure travelers' aspirations and motivations*. Washington, DC: Travel Industry Association.

Devine, J., Camfield, L., & Gough, I. (2008). Autonomy or dependence—Or both?: Perspectives from Bangladesh. *Journal of Happiness Studies, 9*(1), 105–138.

Doherty, W. J. (1999). *How therapy can be hazardous to your marital health*. Paper presented at the Smart Marriages Conference, Washington, DC. Retrieved on September 13, 2016, from www.smartmarriages.com/hazardous.html

Edwards, W., & Milton, M. (2014). Retirement therapy? Older people's experiences of existential therapy relating to their transition to retirement. *Counselling Psychology Review, 29*(2), 43–53.

Fowers, B. J. (2000). *Beyond the myth of marital happiness: How embracing the virtues of loyalty, generosity, justice, and courage can strengthen your relationship*. San Francisco, CA: Jossey-Bass.

Fowers, B. J. (2005). Psychotherapy, character, and the good Life. In B. D. Slife, J. S. Reber, F. C. Richardson, B. D. Slife, J. S. Reber, & F. C. Richardson (Eds.), *Critical thinking about psychology: Hidden assumptions and plausible alternatives* (pp. 39–59). Washington, DC: American Psychological Association.

Fowers, B. J., Richardson, F., & Slife, B. (2017). *Human frailty, vice, and suffering: Flourishing in the context of limits and dependency.* Washington, DC: APA Books.

Fowers, B. J., Tredinnick, M., & Applegate, B. (1997). Individualism and counseling: An empirical examination of the prevalence of individualistic values in psychologists' responses to case vignettes. *Counseling and Values, 41*(3), 204–218. doi:10.1002/j.2161-007X.1997.tb00403.x

Fromm, E. (1941). *Escape from freedom.* New York: Farrar & Rinehart.

Fuscaldo, D. (2012). *10 steps to get you ready for retirement.* Retrieved on September 23, 2016, from www.aarp.org/work/social-security/info-05-2011/10-steps-to-retire-every-day.html

Guignon, C. B. (2004). *On being authentic.* London: Routledge.

Heidegger, M. (1977). *The question concerning technology, and other essays.* New York: Harper & Row.

Heidegger, M., Macquarrie, J., & Robinson, E. (1962). *Being and time.* Malden, MA: Blackwell.

Ingerson, M., DeTienne, K. B., & Liljenquist, K. A. (2015). Beyond instrumentalism: A relational approach to negotiation. *Negotiation Journal, 31*(1), 31–46. doi:10.1111/nejo.12078

Jennings, L., Sovereign, A., Bottorff, N., Mussell, M. P., & Vye, C. (2005). Nine ethical values of master therapists. *Journal of Mental Health Counseling, 27*(1), 32.

Kim, U., Yang, K., & Hwang, K. (Eds.). (2006). *Indigenous and culture psychology: Understanding people in context.* New York, NY: Springer Science+Business Media.

Koole, S. L., & Veenstra, L. (2015). Does emotion regulation occur only inside people's heads? Toward a situated cognition analysis of emotion-regulatory dynamics. *Psychological Inquiry, 26*(1), 61–68. doi:10.1080/1047840X.2015.964657

Kurzban, R., Burton-Chellew, M. N., & West, S. A. (2015). The evolution of altruism in humans. *Annual Review of Psychology, 66,* 575–599. doi:10.1146/annurev-psych-010814-015355

Locke, E. A. (2002). Setting goals for life and happiness. In C. R. Snyder, S. J. Lopez, C. R. Snyder, & S. J. Lopez (Eds.), *Handbook of positive psychology* (pp. 299–312). New York: Oxford University Press.

Marsh, A. A. (2016). Neural, cognitive, and evolutionary foundations of human altruism. *Wires Cognitive Science, 7*(1), 59–71. doi:10.1002/wcs.1377

Meehl, P. E. (1959). Some technical and axiological problems in the therapeutic handling of religious and valuational material. *Journal of Counseling Psychology, 6*(4), 255–259.

Nelson, J. M., & Slife, B. D. (2016). A new positive psychology: A critique of the movement based on early Christian thought. *The Journal of Positive Psychology,* 1–9.

Ostenson, J. A. (2010). Measuring relationships or measuring individuals: An ontological analysis of marital therapy outcome measures. *Dissertation Abstracts International, 71,* 1369.

Oyserman, D., Sorensen, N., Reber, R., & Chen, S. X. (2009). Connecting and separating mind-sets: Culture as situated cognition. *Journal of Personality and Social Psychology, 97*(2), 217–235. doi:10.1037/a0015850

Richardson, F. (2005). Critical thinking about psychology: Hidden assumptions and plausible alternatives. In B. Slife, J. Reber, & F. Richardson (Eds.), *Psychotherapy and modern dilemmas* (pp. 17–38). Washington, DC: American Psychological Association.

Richardson, F. C., Fowers, B. J., & Guignon, C. B. (1999). *Re-envisioning psychology: Moral dimensions of theory and practice.* San Francisco: Jossey-Bass.

Rieff, P. (2006). *The triumph of the therapeutic.* Wilmington, DE: ISI Books (Original work published 1966).

Rogers, C. R. (1951). *Client centred therapy.* Boston: Houghton-Mifflin Co.

Ryan, R. M., & Deci, E. L. (2000). Self-determination theory and the facilitation of intrinsic motivation, social development, and well-being. *American Psychologist, 55*(1), 68–78.

Rychlak, J. F. (1976). *Dialectic: Humanistic rationale for behavior and development.* Basel: Karger.

Rychlak, J. F. (1981). *Introduction to personality and psychotherapy: A theory-construction approach.* Oxford, UK: Houghton Mifflin.

Seligman, M. P. (2011). *Flourish: A visionary new understanding of happiness and well-being.* New York, NY: Free Press.

Skipper International. (2013, May). *Men are happier in retirement than women.* Retrieved from www.skiptoninternational.com/news/men-happier

Slife, B. D. (2015, August). *Liberal individualism: The generic worldview of western psychotherapists.* Paper presented at the meeting of the American Psychological Association, Toronto, Canada.

Slife, B. D. (2016). *The experiencing and theorizing of love.* Paper presented at the meeting of the American Psychological Association, Denver, CO.

Slife, B. D., Koltko, V., & Prows, G. (2013, February). *Relational existential psychotherapy.* Invited address to the United States Air Force mental health staff, Wright-Patterson Air Force Base, Dayton, Ohio.

Slife, B. D., Scott, L., & McDonald, A. (2016). The clash of liberal individualism and theism in psychotherapy: A case illustration. *Open Theology, 2*(1), 596–604. doi:10.1515/opth-2016-0047

Slife, B. D., Smith, A. F., & Burchfield, C. M. (2003). Psychotherapists as crypto-missionaries: An exemplar on the crossroads of history, theory, and philosophy. In D. B. Hill, M. J. Kral, D. B. Hill, & M. J. Kral (Eds.), *About psychology: Essays at the crossroads of history, theory, and philosophy* (pp. 55–69). Albany, NY: State University of New York Press.

Slife, B. D., & Williams, R. (1995). *What's behind the research: Discovering hidden assumptions in the behavioral sciences.* Thousand Oaks, CA: Sage Publications.

Smith, E. R., & Semin, G. R. (2007). Situated social cognition. *Current Directions in Psychological Science, 16*(3), 132–135. doi:10.1111/j.1467–8721.2007.00490.x

Smith, F. M., & Dougherty, D. S. (2012). Revealing a master narrative: Discourses of retirement throughout the working life cycle. *Management Communication Quarterly, 26*(3), 453–478. doi:10.1177/0893318912438687

Society of Counseling Psychology. (2016). *What is counseling psychology.* Retrieved September 15, 2016, from www.div17.org/about-cp/what-is-counseling-psychology/

Szymanski, L. S. (2000). Happiness as a treatment goal. *American Journal on Mental Retardation, 105*(5), 352–362. doi:10.1352/0895-8017(2000)105<0352:HAATG> 2.0.CO;2

Tartakovsky, M. (2016). Therapists spill: How therapy is different from talking to a friend. *Psych Central.* Retrieved on September 10, 2016, from http://psychcentral.com/lib/therapists-spill-how-therapy-is-different-from-talking-to-a-friend/

Tjeltveit, A. C. (1999). *Ethics and values in psychotherapy.* Florence, KY: Taylor & Frances/Routledge.

Tjeltveit, A. C. (2006). To what ends? Psychotherapy goals and outcomes, the good life, and the principle of beneficence. *Psychotherapy: Theory, Research, Practice, Training, 43*(2), 186–200. doi:10.1037/0033-3204.43.2.186

Tredinnick, M. G., & Fowers, B. J. (1999). Individualism and psychotherapy: Are psychologists leading or following individualistic trends? *Counselling Psychology Quarterly, 12*(3), 303–313. doi:10.1080/09515079908254100

4 A Prominent Worldview of Psychological Research

Kari A. O'Grady and Brent D. Slife

The notion that worldviews influence the theoretical expectations and biases of researchers is generally understood in psychological science. In fact, several research procedures are designed to guard against such influences creeping into our results (e.g., experimental controls). Lesser known may be the idea that not only do personal worldviews (e.g. personal culture, beliefs, values, etc.) influence the theoretical biases and expectations of researchers, but that the field of psychology itself has adopted worldview perspectives about psychological science that influence researchers' biases, expectations, and interpretations of the data. Stretching this notion further is the proposal that worldviews influence the investigative methods themselves.

Researchers are in the practice of critiquing one another about the correct deployment of the logic of psychology's methods (e.g., experimental design, replication), but they are virtually unpracticed when it comes to critiquing the fundamental logic of method itself. It is almost as if on some level we believe that the logic of methods is an axiomatic or given that we use to investigate the non-givenness of our hypotheses. It is easy to forget that the logic behind psychology's methods did not present itself in one momentous Big Bang; this logic was developed, defined, and influenced over time by the worldviews of influential scientific figures throughout history.

The primary point of this chapter, then, is to encourage the practice of researcher reflexivity about the influence of worldviews in psychology's research methods, *including* the logic behind the methods. We will demonstrate the value of the dialectic (see Chapter 3) for developing this kind of reflexivity by comparing a prominent worldview influence (WI) in psychological science, naturalism, with that of an alternative, frequently considered non-scientific worldview. The intent is not to promote one worldview over the other, nor is it to point to the limitations of the worldviews, but rather to sensitize researchers to WI in psychological science. We first consider briefly the more familiar WI in research that are outside of method, what is sometimes called the context of discovery (e.g., formulating theory and hypotheses), but the majority of the chapter is spent on the less known WI research influences "inside" the logic of method, what some label as the context of justification (e.g., testing theory and hypotheses).

Worldview Influences Outside of Method

I (O'Grady) teach research methods courses and frequently serve as a methodologist on quantitative and qualitative dissertation studies. Occasionally, students wishing to conduct grounded theory qualitative studies will attempt to convince me that they should not immerse themselves too deeply in the literature or they will be unduly influenced by previous theories and findings which will bias their data collection process. To which I reply that it is not possible for them to empty their brains of theories and worldview influences: their choice of topic and methodology are inevitably informed by theory and reflect biases. Their expectations about what they will find is currently being influenced by their grandmother's philosophies, internet blogs, professors' positions, and childhood experiences, to name just a few such influences. I explain that I would like their biases and expectations to also be informed by theory formulated in their professional field. They then head off to spend the next several months reviewing the literature.

What I am explaining to my students, with most methodologists in agreement, is that it is not possible to engage in research with an empty, unbiased mind. In fact, we could not even begin to ask the questions that inform our hypotheses or guide our research strategies if we approached any topic of human experience without a priori expectations about what we might find. Those expectations are informed by our personal and professional worldviews and what those worldviews tell us about the nature of humans. If, for example, a person's worldview included the view that humans are social beings that are capable of altruistic acts, they would probably be more inclined to form hypotheses that explore questions about social support constructs than someone who views humans as self-contained entities with primarily hedonistic motives. These two types of researchers would then interpret their data and formulate theories based on their distinct views of the nature of humans.

For the most part, modern psychological researchers have some awareness of the influence of culture and personal worldviews on research, but tend to be less aware of the worldview influences that are endemic to psychology itself, such as the professional values of individualism demonstrated in the previous chapter. For example, some researchers may assume that the basic unit of their investigation is the individual, with observations needed for each individual involved. These observations can then, of course, be added together because the assumption is that their individualist, and thus relatively independent, nature allows them to be added together, etc. A relational researcher, by contrast, might assume that the "between-ness" of persons is the fundamental unit of study, with some instrument needed to assess these relationships. If, too, these relationships are themselves related (non-independent), then other statistics might be required to analyze the data.

The point is not that one worldview or investigation is better or more useful. The point is that most methodologists recognize that we need to keep in mind these WI in order to evaluate the research. Unfortunately, because WI are often viewed as "biases" or "values," they are frequently considered potential distortions to objective data and are thus not reported or perhaps even hidden because they embarrass the researcher. Also unfortunate, for similar reasons, is the WI on journal editors and reviewers. Relational reviewers, for instance, could criticize the adding together of individual observations because these reviewers are biased against an individualist worldview without necessarily knowing it (or the reverse)! Without clear awareness and recognition of these WI, both in the formulation of studies and in their evaluation, many research reports could be rejected through sheer, but perhaps unconscious WI. We need to remind ourselves that theoretical conceptions (e.g., topics chosen, hypotheses developed) stem from a worldview, which means that these conceptions of psychology could have been shaped in a different way had another set of worldviews more powerfully influenced the development of the field. Rather than approaching our research with the assumption that our methods can somehow sterilize WI, some argue that scholarly rigor is better achieved by acknowledging that we "approach our subject matter with presuppositions and expectations and are explicit and accountable in that process" as we carry out our research and make our research claims (Jones, 1994, p. 186).

Worldview Influences Inside of Method

As mentioned, most psychologists were taught that if we are not rigorous in our research, the biases and perspectives of our personal worldviews could influence our results (e.g., demand characteristics). We spent valuable and countless hours learning methods for protecting against and accounting for these influences. Most of us, however, are less familiar with the idea that the logic behind the methods of psychological science is based, to some degree at least, on untested WI. This idea is more provocative because most psychological researchers consider the logic of their methods "scientific" and thus neutral to or invisible in the outcome of their research (Slife, Reber, & Faulconer, 2012).

However, psychological science as it is currently conceptualized did not spring forth full-blown from nothing, but has been shaped by the culture, preferences, geographical locations, and values of scholarly social structures over time. Even the logic behind the research, regardless of the method (e.g., experimental, correlational, qualitative), was created by humans over time who themselves were part of cultures with worldviews. Consequently, we need to take into account these WI from the past that are now embodied in our method logic—the context of justification or testing of our ideas—as well as the better known WI that surface in the present—as embodied in the context of discovery or formulation of our ideas. The case for the former, the lesser known WI, make up the bulk of this chapter.

An Amalgam of Worldview Influences

Psychological methods were formulated over time and involve a number of cultural and philosophical influences, including religion, positivism, and secularism. However, we do not have the space to deal with all of them here. Instead, we want to single out one particular influence widely acknowledged outside of psychology—the influence of naturalism. In this manner, we hope to raise the reader's consciousness of WI in research more generally. We are *not* interested in eliminating such influences, partly because conventional methods are fairly successful and partly because this elimination is impossible. Worldview influences are inescapable, regardless of the method. Because the world has not yet been investigated, at least before the formulation of a method, the formulator must make some presumptions (educated guesses) about the world in which the method is deployed in order to think it might be successful (in that world). These WI may not be recognized at the time of this formulation, but they are there nevertheless, and they can originate from one or several cultural or professional sources (e.g., the paradigms of Kuhn, 1970).

The two main sources of WI in regard to psychological methods, at least in the West, are naturalism and theism. It is no coincidence that these two worldviews are also considered the most influential to Western culture generally (Smith, 2001). Much like Western culture writ large, these two great worldviews have etched their impact on psychology's methodology. However, *unlike* other aspects of Western culture, naturalism—through the Enlightenment—has become far more dominant in psychology's methods. We do not have the space here to do a history lesson (Ferngren, 2002; Leahey, 1991), but suffice it to say that the secularism of psychology has led its historical parents to favor the West's naturalistic rather than theistic roots, even though there are also many, hidden influences of theism in the discipline's methods (Delaney & DiClemente, 2005). Consequently, we hope first to describe the influence of this naturalistic worldview and then provide a few examples of its impact on the often taken-for-granted logic of psychological methods. To highlight these WI we contrast them to the other influential worldview of Western culture—theism. We recognize that theism is typically viewed as outside the context of science entirely, but that's precisely the point of its contrast—what worldview assumptions, and thus logic of inquiry, are inside and outside science and what justifies their inclusion?

This type of contrast is considered a kind of dialectic (see Chapter 3). When referring to the dialectic we are not only describing a way of understanding through contrasts and paradoxes, but also suggesting that a thing—a worldview in this case—only actually exists as that thing when there is something other than it to which it can be compared. In other words, many aspects of naturalism are so endemic to psychology's methods that they are not understood or even recognized to exist *as* a WI. By analogy, there is only female because there is male; otherwise female would just be "human." If all humans were female, there would be no need for the idea of female, because it would simply be human. And yet, the human would be comprised of what we in a world of contrasting sexes would view as distinctly female features. So the dialectic exposes the thing to itself.

To carry this analogy just a bit further, the less dominant sex, in our case the less dominant worldview, has historically had to exert a lot of effort trying to convince the more dominant sex that he is not the definition of human, with females as a lesser (or non) expression of human. Interestingly, however, that dialectical effort, the effort of contrasting meanings, has made the female keenly aware of the male. The male on the other hand has fewer pressures to justify his humanness and thus is typically less awareness that he is only one and not the primary expression of human. He will likely need to make deliberate efforts to dialectically expose his assumptions and biases about his definition of human to increase his awareness of what makes him the male expression of human. But what has all of this discussion of the sexes and expression of humanness got to do with psychological science and worldviews? Isn't science just science?

In dialectically comparing naturalism to theism, we recognize that theists are not typically understood to be knowledge advancers, but theists do advance, after a fashion, the knowledge of their interest—scripture meanings, God's attributes, and even divine influences in the natural world. They just do not advance knowledge in the currently accepted manner of psychological science. One could argue that what is currently accepted as the logic of psychological is a product of valid evolutionary processes in the formulation of psychology methods, separating the naturalistic wheat from the theistic chaff. Again, however, our purpose here is not to argue that theism should be included in the canon of psychological methods.

We just want to use theism to highlight various aspects of methodological naturalism.[1] Much like the female aids the male in understanding his status as human, theism's outsider status in psychological science can help us to understand naturalism's insider status—the logic of conventional method—better.

As was the case in Chapter 3, we wish to avoid awkward phrasing as we contrast worldview influences in research. In this chapter we use the terms "naturalist" and "theist" as shorthand for a person who is currently seeing the world from or acting on a particular worldview perspective. We do not mean to preclude the possibility, as we use these terms, that actual whomever uses worldviews either can mix worldviews or apply them situationally by relying more upon one than another in any particular context.

The Worldview of Naturalism

Naturalism is frequently defined in a twofold manner—its abdication of the supernatural (e.g., God) and its affirmation of the notion that objective natural laws govern the world. Theists would obviously disagree with the first part of this definition but it may not be well known that they would *not* necessarily disagree with the second. In other words, most naturalists and theists believe and are interested in the regularities, patterns, or "laws" of the natural world as well as the susceptibility of these regularities to the rationality of human investigation. However, many naturalists and theists might disagree about how the laws work, the meaning of those laws, etc. Consider, for example, Charles Taylor on this point:

> Modern science offers us a view of the universe framed in general laws. The ultimate is an *impersonal* order of regularities in which all particular things exist, over-arching all space and time. This seems *in conflict* with Christian faith, which relates us to a *personal* Creator-God, and which explains our predicament in terms of a developing exchange of divine action and human reaction to his interventions in history.
>
> (p. 362)

This quote from Taylor (italics added) seems to distinguish two very different meanings of order in the two worldviews of naturalism and theism, the first an impersonal, lawful, and determined order, and the second a personal, divine, and obedient order, at least for this particular tradition (Christian) of theism. The point here is that the common term "order" denotes the importance of natural regularities for both worldviews, hence the possibility of some complementary work between researchers from the two worldviews. Still, it must be noted that the nature, source, and meaning of order can be substantially different and could conceivably lead to very different methods and practices, even in considering the "regularities" of the world.

In this sense, there might be many aspects of method in common—due to some common assumptions such as order and rationality—but there are still important aspects that might be different. We focus below on a few differences only to highlight them. We do this, in part, to combat the notion— common among psychological investigators—that the current logic of their method is *completely* neutral to all worldviews. Some aspects, procedures, and strategies of psychological research may not be shared. And, as we will see, these differences can potentially influence every step of the research process: topic selection, methodological approach, research design, selection of items on research measures, and the analysis and interpretation of data.

Worldview Differences in Research

We start with two obviously different WI in this logic involving divine guidance and immanence, and then we describe three more subtle differences: the need for generalization, the need to separate the subjective from the objective, and the need to detect causality.

Obvious Differences

Divine Guidance

Naturalism, of course, does not imply that researchers should pray for divine guidance in their research nor does it presume that God can or should guide the research process. Similar to naturalism, many theists can consider systematic observation an important way to gain knowledge, but they typically do not consider this mode of experience the *only* way to advance knowledge. Many theists, for instance, also presume that God cares about and is involved in all human endeavors, so these theists assume that God can enlighten scientists in their research efforts, if not affect the research itself. The theist may rely on the scientific method while *also* assuming that God's guidance and influence can "get us to some truths that would otherwise be inaccessible to us" (Kemp, 1998, p. 466). Therefore, God is at least a necessary condition for true knowledge advancement, whereas God is irrelevant to the naturalist. Interestingly, many natural and behavioral scientists do report feeling some divine guidance in the context of discovery—the context of formulating their theory and hypotheses. However, these scientists frequently assume that there is no need for prayer or divine guidance in the context of justification—the process of the method's working and testing these theories and ideas (O'Grady & Richards, 2011).

Immanence

Naturalists also confine their studies to the natural world, whereas theists are interested in both the supernatural and natural worlds. However, theists typically do not label the transcendent or divine as "supernatural," because they have no reason to distinguish the two worlds—God is considered to be involved in both. The notion of supernatural is a naturalistic term and conception anyway—understanding what is "super" or beyond the natural requires understanding the natural (Griffin, 2001). Moreover, the naturalist has to understand the natural apart from the supernatural, a dualism or separation that most theists would not endorse. Indeed, theists would likely hold that the natural could not be understood completely without knowledge of the transcendent or divine, given the integration of the two "worlds." In this sense, the worldviews of theists and naturalists allow them both to be interested in the natural world, but only the naturalists assume a dualism that leads them to confine their studies to the natural world exclusively. Some naturalists might contend that such a dualism is not necessary for their naturalistic worldview, because they do not believe the supernatural exists, so there is no need to distinguish the natural from it. This contention, however, would belie a lot of historical and contemporary attempts to demarcate the scientific from the pseudo-scientific in psychology, with much of the latter understood as attempts to access and advance knowledge of the spiritual or transcendent. In any case, the point here is the clear difference between the theistic broadening of the world of interest to include the "supernatural" and the naturalistic reduction of the world to the natural, at least in comparison.

Even these examples of obvious areas of WI difference, divine guidance and immanence, can begin to sharpen our awareness of the influence of worldviews in the logic of psychological methods. Method texts in psychology do not counsel psychological researchers to pray over or seek divine guidance in their experiments, and they do not advise these investigators to formulate procedures for studying the elements of the supernatural—*for worldview reasons*. Again, someone may say that the absence of these practices is because psychology is about "science" and not "religion," but then this assertion merely begs the question of this chapter: why these particular practices in psychological science? There is no more empirical evidence for *not* seeking divine guidance in conducting experiments as there is for seeking it. Indeed, there is no empirical evidence for empiricism itself. These are views of the world or views of knowledge advancement that need to be assumed *before* investigation can occur in order to get the evidence.

Less obvious WI require even closer attention to the taken-for-granted nature of WI. For this reason, the following WI in psychological methods are easily mistaken for the givens or the axioms of research as opposed to the WI that they are. Some psychologists may view the presence of such WI as embarrassing, as if these expose hidden biases and thus vitiate the validity of psychological investigations. Again, however, *there are no methods—in the natural or behavioral sciences—that do not involve WI*. Not only are these worldview influences inescapable; they are necessary to the knowledge gained. Such worldview influences are *inherent to* the method and are not some artifact that should be kept apart from it. Therefore, we need to take them into account as we gather our data and make our interpretations—what we are calling here researcher reflexivity.

Subtle Differences

As mentioned, worldview influences can also be manifested in psychological research in subtler ways. We consider here the psychological investigator's typical need to find generalization, prevent bias, and discover causality.

The Need for Generalization

To discover the natural or social laws assumed by naturalists, generalizable findings are pivotal. Studies that are generalizable are presumed to have the potential to become dependable laws that will manifest consistently across populations. Given the lawfulness of laws, this generalizability implies the importance of other method conceptions, including replication, reliability, standardization, quantification (to help make comparisons), and even the approximation of these laws in less prestigious correlational studies. In fact, generalizability is so influential to psychological methods that non-generalizable (or unique or singular) findings are often considered bogus or unreal (e.g., parapsychology).

Of course, theists would also be interested in generalizable findings, because many of them believe that God created and sustains the regularities and generalities of nature. The difference, however, is that they would not *automatically* reject non-generalizable findings because many forms of knowledge, including many psychological forms of knowledge, from their perspective may only occur once and still have implications for the present and future. This means that some aspects of psychological methods (e.g., replication, standardization, reliability) are not automatically required, and some methods might be devised that attempt to detect uniquenesses and singularities.

Some psychological researchers might argue that such unique events would have no implication transfer to other situations and context, given that they only occurred once and thus have no real psychological relevance for the present or future. However, there are other notions of relevance than the repeatability of a particular pattern of natural events. The Big Bang, for example, is thought to have occurred only once but still has implications for the present and future. Or closer to home for many theists, many religious people have experienced distinctly singular spiritual experiences only once that nevertheless hold vital psychological relevance for them into the future and other situations. The point again is not that one or the other worldview is more correct than the other; the point is that WI are fairly directly affecting some aspects of current psychological methods.

The Need to Separate the Subjective From the Objective

The objectivity of natural laws is also important for the naturalist, because these are the laws of a pristine nature that should be distinguished from the opinions and biases of psychological researchers. Consequently, the real and the meaningful, from a naturalist perspective, are those regularities that are both generalizable (and thus candidates for lawfulness) and objective (not subjective). This separation of the subjective from the objective, another form of dualism, is therefore the prime reason that researcher biases, values, and subjectivity of all sorts in psychological science are considered bad— potential distortions of objective data. This worldview reasoning in our methodology has thus led to all kinds of method procedures from the prevention of demand characteristics to the need for control groups. The irony is that this WI, as we have mentioned, has also led naturalistic researchers to attempt to avoid or ignore WI, because such influences are considered biases and thus distortions of the pristine natural world (and one of the reasons a book like this needs to be written).

Many theists, on the other hand, not only admit to and prize many subjective conceptions, such as spirituality, beliefs, and values, but also hold that many types and pieces of knowledge are only accessible to researchers with the right interpretations and values (e.g., in Christianity, "he who hath ears to hear", and in Judaism, *Shema* "Hear O Israel"). From this frame of reference, hermeneutic qualitative research, which assumes the value and even necessity of the researcher's interpretation in discovering knowledge (e.g., Packer), could be as important as experimental quantitative research to the theist.

Take, for example, Kohlberg's early work on moral development. This research was assumed to objectively measure levels of moral development, with obedience to moral authority reflecting a low level of moral development; blind obedience to a religious leader was considered to undermine the need for complex decision making. However, many theists conceptualize moral authority in a complex system of both divine and human authority. Richards and Davison (1992), for instance, make the case that such complex reasoning requires *more* advanced moral development not less. Given that theists make up the bulk of psychology's clientele, Kohlberg's interpretations and values regarding moral authority may not have been the right interpretations and values to understand the *actual* experience of moral authority and moral development, at least for many theists (see Richards & Davison, 1992).

The Need to Detect Causality

Physical or psychological laws are also thought to be "causal" laws for the naturalist. That is, the naturalist assumes that natural laws govern the entities of the world, including humans, and thus discovering the causation of this governance is important to understanding the laws themselves. This feature of naturalism is one of the reasons that experimental design is the most highly prized method logic in psychological research; it supposedly provides evidence for and an understanding of this causality, and thus how the physical or psychological laws govern nature.

Again, this type of research could also be important to the theist, given their interest in the regularities of nature, but many theists also assume human agency, which would presume that humans are not governed or caused (or determined) by natural laws but rather are more constrained by them. Many theists, for example, assume that in order for humans to love others and God, they must have the capacity, at least to some degree, to choose to do otherwise. Without this capacity, their love would be no different from other entities governed by natural laws, such as a boulder rolling down a mountain, and this "love" would thus not be meaningful. Experimental evidence, from this theistic perspective of human agency, is not necessarily the most important type of evidence.

Indeed, this evidence might be viewed as inappropriate for some types of specifically human phenomena. Some psychology of religion researchers, for example, have attempted to use experimental methods for understanding sanctification (Pargament & Mahoney, 2005), but others have argued that this approach strips away what sanctification actually is—the use of one's agency to engage in a sacred relationship with God through the dedication of one's will in service of that relationship. The point again is that the assumption of causal law, and thus the need to detect it, has led the naturalist to a particular approach to method that other worldviews do not necessarily need to hold.

Can Theists Use Naturalist Method Features?

The short answer to this question is yes. Not only are there method features in common, such as order and rationality, theists should feel free to explore strategies and approaches to methods that are considered to be more manifestations of naturalism, even in the service of their worldviews (just as naturalists might probe into distinctly theistic features). The obvious caveat to these uses is that researchers should become sensitive to the possible influences of worldviews that may complement or detract from the goals of their investigations. From a theist perspective, for example, researchers should not be locked into knowledge gathering that exclusively investigates replicable, objective, or causal phenomena, even if much of this knowledge gathering could be relevant to the theist. To be "locked in," given the logic of conventional psychological methods, is to be guided both in *what* is investigated and in *how* it is investigated, which is to "make a metaphysic of the method," as Burtt (2003) warned so many years ago. In other words, without suitable awareness, the method itself can affect the results in ways that the researcher has no knowledge.

From the perspective of WI, such method biases cannot be avoided, because all methods are human-created and thus implicitly entail an amalgam of the worldviews of the humans involved. However, this human involvement does not mean that researchers with worldviews other than those entailed in the methods cannot use them. A carpenter can skillfully use a hammer to pound a screw—a connector not designed for hammer pounding—but the good carpenter bears in mind the pros and cons of such a connector when it has undergone such pounding. Moreover, theism was itself historically involved in the formulation of scientific method, which means it has its own features endemic to psychological methods. Our contrast of naturalism and theism here is only meant to highlight some of the naturalistic method features of psychological methods. It is not meant to rule out such features for the skillful and careful use of theists, as we have noted throughout this chapter.

***

The aim of this chapter was to encourage the practice of researcher reflexivity about WI in psychological science. Many researchers have developed a level of sensitivity to WI in formulating and evaluating research, but most are less aware of the need to attend to WI in the logic behind the research methods themselves. They may have assumed that previous researchers have tested this logic through some evolution of their repeated and seemingly successful use, yet there is no historical evidence that they have system-atically tested this method logic against *other* logics of methods. And even if researchers wanted to compare logics of method, what logic of method would they use to do the comparison? Our point is a simple one: all methods are based to some degree on untested worldviews, views of the world in which the methods would likely be successful.

We also used the time-tested dialectic to encourage researcher reflexivity by highlighting WI in the logic of methods. We chose one of the well-known WI in the West—theism—to help elucidate psychology's prominent WI: natural-ism. Theism's outsider status qualified it to expose the "thing"—naturalism—to itself. Once again, the point of comparing the two WIs was not to claim that one worldview or method of investigation is better or more useful, but rather to increase researchers' sensitivity to the influence of worldviews in in the taken-for-granted expectations of psychological science.

One of those expectations is that researchers should not reach beyond the evidence in their claim by drawing conclusions about the findings without accounting for additional influences on the results. We are, for example, expected to use methods to attend to possible historical influences in our longitudinal studies or other potential cofounds (e.g., social desirability) in our research. In other words, the logic behind our methods, itself likely influenced by a worldview, requires us to justify our claims by considering a variety of possible influences in our findings. Attending to and account-ing for these influences helps researchers to avoid making claims about the world without recognizing the embedded, and perhaps even long-forgotten, cultural views influencing their method logic.

Note

1 We understand that some have argued for a fairly sharp dividing line between methodological and metaphysical naturalism (e.g., Bishop, 2009). However, we would contend that this line, though important for some purposes, is more blurred in the present context. In this sense, epistemologies such as methodological natu-ralism are influenced by ontologies such as metaphysical naturalism, and vice versa. Hence, we focus here on more of the blurring than the dividing, hoping to avoid the deeper philosophical issues of their relationship (see Slife & Reber, 2012 for more information).

References

Bishop, R. (2009). What is all this naturalism stuff about? *Journal of Theoretical and Philosophical Psychology, 29*, 108–113.

Burtt, E. A. (2003). *The metaphysical foundations of modern science*. Mineola, NY: Dover.

Delaney, H. B., & DiClemente, C. C. (2005). Psychology's roots: A brief history of the influence of Judeo-Christian perspectives. In W. R. Miller & H. D. Delaney

(Eds.), *Judeo-Christian perspectives on psychology*. Washington, DC: American Psychological Association.

Ferngren, G. B. (2002). *Science and religion: A historical introduction*. Baltimore, MD: Johns Hopkins University Press.

Griffin, D. R. (2001). *Reenchantment without supernaturalism: A process philosophy of religion*. Ithaca, NY: Cornell University Press.

Jones, S. L. (1994). A constructive relationship for religion with the science and profession of psychology: Perhaps the boldest model yet. *American Psychologist, 49,* 184–199.

Leahey, T. H. (1991). *A history of modern psychology*. Englewood Cliffs, NJ: Prentice Hall.

Pargament, K. I., & Mahoney, A. (2005). Sacred matters: Sanctification as a vital topic for the psychology of religion, *The International Journal for the Psychology of Religion, 15*(3), 179–198.

Richards, P. S., & Davison, M. L. (1992). Religious bias in moral development research: A psychometric investigation. *Journal for the Scientific Study of Religion, 31*(4), 467–485.

Slife, B. D., Reber, J. S., & Faulconer, J. E. (2012). Implicit ontological reasoning: Problems of dualism in psychological science. *Psychology of science: Implicit and explicit reasoning*. New York: Oxford University Press.

Smith, H. (2001). *Why religion matters*. New York: Harper Collins.

5 Cultures, Worlds, and Worldviews

Louise Sundararajan

Imagine this scenario: On the Cartesian stage, a scientist is conducting an experiment, when all of a sudden the curtain behind her that hides the back-stage is lifted. Lifting the curtain on cross-culture psychology reveals a circular movement which entails one culture studying another culture; or one particular worldview investigating another. To get outside this circularity, the researcher needs to become self-reflexive by acknowledging the world-views of the research culture. Consistent with this call for a self-reflexive turn in psychology (Sundararajan, 2008), this chapter will (1) examine the worldviews behind the Cartesian theater of psychology, with special focus on the worldviews behind a cross cultural study of social cynicism; (2) explore alternative worldviews that give a different account of cynicism; and (3) discuss the implications of this investigation for theory, research, and ethics.

Worldviews of the Cartesian Theater of Science

One hallmark of science on the Cartesian stage is its objectivity which implies that the scientist has no worldviews (see also Chapters 3 and 4 of this volume). But once the curtain is lifted to reveal the back stage, we see that psychology is the product of a particular culture, which has been referred to as primarily WEIRD (Western, Educated, Industrialized, Rich, and Democratic) (Henrich, Heine, & Norenzayan, 2010). The WEIRD worldviews can be adumbrated as follows.

Humans Are Thinkers, Not Agents

Descartes privileges thinking as the defining attribute of being human, in sharp contrast to many other cultures, for instance Confucianism, in which agency is primary. In cross-cultural psychology, the Cartesian legacy may have contributed to an over-abundance of measurements on beliefs.

Cartesian Dualism

In the Cartesian system, the self is not in the world so much as an observer that stands apart from and over against the world (see also Chapter 2). This assumption is a corollary of the supremacy of thinking, as thinking can be disembodied, in sharp contrast to the agent's action which necessarily takes place in the world.

The Individual Psyche

Mainstream psychology is infested with individualism (see Chapter 4). Since the individual is a bonded being with an interior that no one else has access to, the mental life of the individual necessarily takes place inside the individual, leaving the world out in the cold so to speak. For instance, perception is widely considered in psychology as a brain event, an internal processing. Within this framework, the role of affect is to collect evolutionarily relevant information about the world for the brain to make a quick and handy map (representation) of the world. According to Noë (2009), "The world itself . . . just doesn't get into the act. . . . At best. . . . The world causally perturbs the nervous system at its periphery (the senses), thus giving rise to the events that cause us to seem to see" (pp. 136–137).

Mental Life Cast in the Space of Causation

Under the sway of mechanism, the law of causation (see Chapter 3) that governs objects in the material world is extended to the mental life of agents/subjects. This is referred to by Levinas (1973) as the "naturalistic worldview" which "places subject and object in the same world, which it calls nature, and studies their relation as a relation of causality" (p. 15).

For illustration, I examine the worldviews behind a cross-cultural study of worldviews (Chen et al., 2015).

Worldviews Behind a Study of Worldviews

In this cross-cultural study, the authors (Chen et al., 2015) touted the importance of studying worldviews of other cultures. However, when they said that worldviews of other cultures "count," they neglected to count in their own worldviews. In this section, I examine the worldviews behind this study.

Supremacy of Beliefs

Consistent with the Cartesian self as thinker, the researchers focus on beliefs as the royal road to culture. The beliefs they study are social axioms

(Leung & Bond, 2004), in particular the axiom of social cynicism. The cynical belief—mistrust of powerful others and social institutions—derives from perceiving corruption of power and disregard of ethical means to achieve an end. Thus the social cynicism factor consists of items that "represent a negative view of human nature, especially as it is easily corrupted by power, a biased view against some groups of people, a mistrust of social institutions, and a disregard of ethical means for achieving an end" (Leung & Bond, 2004, p. 134). For instance, the following item had the highest loading: "Powerful people tend to exploit others."

Cartesian Dualism

Consistent with Cartesian dualism is the assumption that self and world can be treated as two independent concepts or two discrete units of analysis. Thus by "worldview" the authors (Chen et al., 2015) meant literally view of the world, which is supposed to be a concept separate and distinct from view of the self—the former was measured by social cynicism and the latter, self-esteem.

The Inward Turn to Psyche

The original study of social axioms (Leung & Bond, 2004) was an analysis at the level of nations survey. But the study by Chen et al. (2015), falling prey to individualism that focuses on the individual psyche, has turned social cynicism into a personality trait which impacts on the individual's well-being through another personality variable—self-esteem.

Causal Explanation of Cynicism

According to Leung and Bond's (2004) study of social axioms at the national level, social cynicism was significantly and negatively correlated to life satisfaction, achievement via conformity, and with view on charismatic/value-based leadership, while significantly and positively correlated to the pace of life. Chen et al. (2015) added a few more details to this causal chain of cynicism. For instance, cynicism was found to have negative impact on well-being mainly through negative self-view in the form of comparative self-criticism.

An Alternative Approach to Cynicism

An alternative approach to cynicism is found in the study of a village community in Bashan, China, by the anthropologist Hans Steinmüller (Steinmüller, 2013). The author carefully examines a slew of worldviews in anthropology and selectively espouses a worldview that is informed by humanistic and continental philosophies. The result is a very different presentation of cynicism. In this study of life in contemporary rural China, cynicism is located in the tension between the government and the subaltern, more specifically in that between the public official representations and what goes on in the privacy of the villagers' collective introspection:

> There is a 'coded tension' between official representations, generally linked to nation and state, and vernacular forms in face-to-face communities; this tension expresses itself in embarrassment, *cynicism*, or irony.
>
> (Steinmüller, 2013, p. 23, emphasis added)

Agent in Action

Instead of beliefs, the focus of Steinmüller's (2013) analysis is on persons as agents. Agents act. In this framework, cynicism has to do with the mental action of reflecting on everyday morality, especially at the juncture of its breakdown, for instance, when the government is not fair. A case in point is the government's rural construction program which gave subsidies to remodel or build new houses—only for villagers who lived near the public road, not those whose farms were higher up in the mountains, away from the asphalt road. This is an occasion for cynicism: "I tell you, look at the houses here, off the street: the government doesn't do anything. This fucking reconstruction programme sucks. They serve themselves, and don't serve the people" (p. 232), said one farmer. Cynicism is also expressed in irony. When Steinmüller (2013) confided in his farmer friend his concerns about the fate of his doctoral dissertation, which was to be written on the basis of his field work in Bashan, his friend said that now that Steinmüller had understood how things work in China, nothing would be easier: "Just write long praises of rural development, the good side of the things you saw here. Then get your friends in the university and in the government to publish it. I'm sure you'll do well" (p. 232).

Self in the World

Heidegger claims that being is being in the world. From this point of view, cynicism reveals a particular self-world relation. More specifically, cynicism marks the agent's marginality in social standing, a marginality steeped in feelings of powerlessness—and embarrassment (Steinmüller, 2013). This may explain why social cynicism is associated with low well-being scores, and low self-esteem, especially in the form of comparative self-criticism, in the study of Chen et al. (2015). However, from the Heideggerian point of view, these statistical correlations with measures of the individual psyche, such as self-esteem and happiness, should not distract from the more important function of cynicism as an index of self-world relation.

From Individual to Community

One important contribution of Steinmüller's (2013) study is that it shows how beyond (negative) individual thinking and feeling, cynicism serves the (positive) function in forming group solidarity. When he was told by the villagers, "finally you have understood how propaganda works here and what the rural reconstruction programmes are all about" (p. 232), Steinmüller knew that he was now an insider of the "communities of complicity." By "communities of complicity" Steinmüller refers to "communities of those 'in the know', those who share an experiential horizon and an intimate knowledge" (p. 224). This intimate knowledge, otherwise referred to as "cultural intimacy," consists of "the self-recognition of people who are aware that what is dear and important to them is corrupt, backwards, and potentially embarrassing to outsiders" (p. 223). While consistent with what Chen et al. (2015) refer to as low self-esteem stemming from comparative self-criticism, this embarrassment of the villagers serves a positive purpose at the level of collective introspection. Steinmüller (2013) has documented extensively how indirect expressions and action such as embarrassment, cynicism, and irony opened up "an intimate space of common knowledge" (p. 220), thereby forming the basis for a community. In this community, "Covertness, embarrassment, cynicism, and irony are communicative strategies that make it possible to acknowledge both sides of the contradiction, to avoid confrontation, and to maintain communication" (p. 22). Such a community of complicity serves well the purpose of those who subsist on the margin of the ever more progressive society of modern China.

From the Space of Causation to the Space of Reasons

Steinmüller's (2013) study of the "community of complicity" challenges the causal interpretation of social cynicism as formulated by Leung and Bond (2004, p. 166): "People high in social cynicism seem unable to cope with their social world effectively, resulting in considerable negative psychological outcomes." The problem with causal explanations of human behavior is that it eliminates human agency, as Brinkmann (2006, p. 5) points out. By defining humans as agents, Steinmüller's (2013) study locates mental life not in the space of causation so much as in the space of reasons (Brinkmann, 2006). This paradigm shift has far-reaching consequences.

First as agents who act, the individual is necessarily engaged with the world. As Brinkmann (2006) points out, "The normative reasons for action, feeling and thought that we are faced with are *not* as such *psychological properties of the agent* (e.g. desires or representations), but aspects of our world of human interaction and social practices" (p. 12, emphasis added). This means, for our purposes, that social cynicism is not a personality trait so much as an index of the agent's engagement with the world. To understand cynicism as the agent's engagement with the world is to situate it in the agent's discursive practices of giving and receiving reasons for actions.

Agents are concerned with normative reasons for action. Brinkmann (2006) uses anger to explain this point. "What makes 'boiling of the blood' *anger* is not something found in the blood, but precisely that it is situated in a practical context where it makes sense to question, justify and state the reason for 'boiling of the blood'" (p. 5). Substitute *anger* for *cynicism*, and we arrive at an account of social cynicism as behavior driven not by causal so much as normative necessity: Cynicism is a manifestation of the collective introspection in which the villagers question, justify, and state the reason for the gap between the official representations and their private norms.

What are being questioned in the discourse called cynicism? Holiday (1988) has identified three pre-conventional, not socially constructed, values that lie at the core of all language-games: truth-telling, justice, and ritual. All three of these basic human values were questioned by the villagers of Bashan—the government's failure in truth-telling and justice is the source of their cynicism and irony, while their own rituals of gift giving, gambling, and so on are the source of their embarrassment (to outsiders such as government). Far from being simply subjective feelings of low self-esteem and unhappiness, social cynicism is concerned with the most basic questions of morality—as Steinmüller (2013) points out that when awkwardness and irony are put into action, they "imply a properly ethical stance: a reflective engagement with moral frameworks" (p. 228).

Implications for Theory and Research

> "We don't see things as they are, we see them as we are."
> (Anaïs Nin, cited in Chen et al., 2015, p. 762)

How Many Worlds Are There Behind Worldviews?

Approaching cultures as worldviews runs the risk of reducing different cultures to different views on presumably one and the same world. But so far as mental life is concerned, different cultures are literally different worlds (Sundararajan, 2015). Shweder (1991) puts it this way: "It is a supposition of cultural psychology that when people live in the world differently, it maybe that they live in *different worlds*. It is an appreciation of those *different worlds* that cultural psychology tries to achieve" (p. 23, emphasis added). Shweder goes on to spell out the consequences of this formulation of culture: If cultures disagree, "They are not contradictions battling with each other in the same world. They are arguments in different worlds . . . When you live in the same world all disagreements are matters of error, ignorance, or misunderstanding. When you live in different worlds there is far more to a disagreement than meets the eye" (p. 18). In order to understand the worlds behind worldviews, we do well to consult Martin Heidegger.

Heidegger (1971) claims that "a stone is worldless. Plant and animal likewise have no world. . . . The peasant woman, on the other hand, has a world" (p. 45). But what is it to have a world? In answering this question, Heidegger invites us to contemplate a Greek temple that stands "in the middle of the rock-cleft valley" (p. 41). The temple:

> gathers around itself the unity of those paths and relations in which birth and death, disaster and blessing, victory and disgrace, endurance and decline acquire the shape of destiny for human being. The all-governing expanse of this open relational context is the *world* of this historical people.
>
> (p. 42, emphasis added)

As this example suggests, art work (such as the temple) has the power to open up a world. But wait, doesn't the worldview of the artist gives shape to art which in turn opens a world? This is getting things backward, says Heidegger. First of all, consider art work in a museum. Museum art cannot open a world, because it is decontextualized. The world-opening power of the art work comes from its embeddedness in its culture as a living reality, or as Heidegger puts it, the living reality of a world is there so long as the god has not fled from the temple:

> The temple, in its standing there, first gives to things their look and to men their outlook on themselves [e.g., self-views]. This view remains open as long as the [art] work is a work, as long as the god has not fled from it.
>
> (p. 43)

Only then, those who inhabit in that world can derive from it a particular worldview or a particular outlook on things and on themselves. From this point view, cultures are lived-worlds that make worldviews possible, but cannot be reduced to worldviews without losing vitally important information for the research.

From Causal to Normative Necessity

The canonical worldviews of mainstream psychology can result in wasting our time "doing experiments to demonstrate causal connections between elements (e.g. unexpected stimuli and surprise) that are already normatively (i.e., conceptually) connected" (Brinkmann, 2006, p. 5). A case in point is the study by Chen et al. (2015) which found, after a series of analysis with much statistical rigor, that "inherent in self-views are not only schematic representations of internal attributes but also mental convictions about external contexts" (p. 759). So view of the self and view of the world are actually inextricably connected! Is this a real discovery of the mind that no one with common sense could have figured out on their own? Or is it a revelation only to those who have been caught in the trap of the Cartesian self-world dualism?

Besides creating methodological blind alleys, worldviews in mainstream psychology can also have negative impact on people's lives, through a process called psychologization.

Psychologization

Overspill of psychological signifiers is known as psychologization, which is defined by De Vos (2012) as "psychological vocabulary and psychological explanatory schemes entering fields which are supposed not to belong to the traditional theoretical and practical terrains of psychology" (p. 1). Psychologization has far-reaching consequences on people's lives. As we are acting and self-interpreting beings—a phenomenon referred to by Hacking (1995) as the looping effects of human kinds—the researchers' understandings can enter the loop of people's self-understanding. Consequently, as Brinkmann (2006) points out: "Researchers can assist in inventing new forms of mental life, sometimes in valuable ways (cf. the history of feminist research), but sometimes in questionable ways" (p. 7). One form of mental life promoted by the Chinese government, with the help of imported psychology, centers around happiness and well-being.

The recent psycho-boom in China—marked by importing psychology, especially positive psychology, whole sale—has been well documented by Jie Yang (2015). Ever since China downsized and privatized its state-owned enterprises, psychology has played an important role in state-led interventions to alleviate the effects of mass layoff and unemployment. Leaders of state enterprises suggest that the only efficient way to deal with unemployment is to help laid-off workers to "acquire the value structure that leads to positive self-esteem and self-sufficiency for the market economy" (p. 41). Thus, as the laid-off workers were being counseled and reoriented to the market economy, promotion of happiness and well-being has become the nation's top priority. Critics refer to this phenomenon as psychologization, which is defined by Yang (2015) as "socioeconomic issues . . . managed in 'psychological' modes of thinking" (p. 6). Yang (2015) argues that the programs that promote happiness and positive psychology "attempt to provide psychological solutions to social issues" (p. 37). More specifically, "By turning economic stratification into personal, emotional, and psychological conditions, happiness promotions downplayed structural inequalities" (p. 58).

The Chinese laid-off workers are also not too excited about psychologization, except that they use cynicism and irony instead to get their point across. One popular Chinese saying captures well their negativity: "When those at the top are sick, why must those at the bottom be given medicine?" (p. 1). At one training session for the laid-off workers, the director of the reemployment service center emphasized the importance of optimism: "Those who beam with optimism and smile will get hired first. That's why you need to be optimistic. No employer likes a person who is bitter or grumpy" (p. 55). One worker who attended the session remarked, "Most jobs we can apply for are dirty labor work. No one wants to shake hands with you or see how big your smile is. It's hard to smile, considering the way we have been treated [laid off]" (p. 55). But irony shall have the last word. According to Yang (2015), the counseling client used "irony to reject, resist, or even integrate psychologization" (p. 74). The following exchange (p. 75) shall suffice as an example:

> The job counselor: "Unemployment at least gives you an opportunity for a new beginning, which can mean entrepreneurship."
> One laid-off worker: "What kind of entrepreneurship? An entrepreneur who drinks wind from the Northwest? [having nothing to eat but wind from Siberia, meaning cold and hungry]."

In conclusion, different worldviews serve different purposes for the researcher. A reductionist approach, used for instance in multi-nations survey on beliefs, is good for cross-cultural comparison on demographics, such as religion, economics, power structure, population, mortality, and so on. However, to understand the culturally different Other it is necessary, for reasons adumbrated in the foregoing analysis, to approach cultures as lived worlds that cannot be reduced to beliefs or worldviews.

References

Brinkmann, S. (2006). Mental life in the space of reasons. *Journal for the Theory of Social Behavior, 36*, 1–16.

Chen, S. X., Lam, B. C. P., Wu, W. C. H., Ng, J. C. K., Buchtel, E. E., Guan, Y., & Deng, H. (2015). Do people's world views matter? The why and how. *Journal of Personality and Social Psychology, 110*, 743–765.

De Vos, J. (2012). *Psychologisation in times of globalisation*. London, UK: Routledge.

Hacking, I. (1995). The looping effect of human kinds. In D. Sperber, D. Premack, & A. J. Premack (Eds.), *Causal cognition: A multidisciplinary debate* (pp. 351–383). Oxford: Clarendon Press.

Heidegger, M. (1971). *Poetry, language, thought* (Albert Hofstadter, Trans.). New York, NY: Harper & Row.

Henrich, J., Heine, S. J., & Norenzayan, A. (2010). The weirdest people in the world? *Behavioral and Brain Sciences, 33*, 61–83.

Holiday, A. (1988). *Moral powers: Normative necessity in language and history*. London: Routledge.

Leung, K., & Bond, M. (2004). Social axioms: A model for social beliefs in multicultural perspective. *Advances in Experimental Social Psychology, 36*, 122–199.

Levinas, E. (1973). *The theory of intuition in Husserl's phenomenology*. Evanston, IL: Northwestern University Press.

Noë, A. (2009). *Out of our heads*. New York, NY: Hill and Wang.

Shweder, R. A. (1991). *Thinking through culture: Expeditions in cultural psychology*. Cambridge, MA: Harvard University Press.

Steinmüller, H. (2013). *Communities of complicity: Everyday ethics in rural China*. New York, NY: Berghahn.

Sundararajan, L. (2008). Toward a reflexive positive psychology: Insights from the Chinese Buddhist notion of emptiness. In J. C. Christopher, F. C. Richardson, & B. D. Slife (Eds.), Thinking through positive psychology, a special issue of *Theory & Psychology, 18*, 655–674.

Sundararajan, L. (2015). *Understanding emotion in Chinese culture: Thinking through psychology*. New York, NY: Springer SBM.

Yang, J. (2015). *Unknotting the heart: Unemployment and therapeutic governance in China*. Ithaca, NY: Cornell University Press.

6 Toward Worldview Pluralism in Psychology

Russell D. Kosits

With great love, I dedicate this chapter to my father, Roger A. Kosits, who struggled with and died from lung cancer during the time this chapter was written. He was a tolerant man and, I trust, would have sympathized with the pluralistic ideals expressed herein.

* * *

Human beings are powerfully shaped—and divided—by their worldviews, or beliefs about ultimate questions. Implicitly or explicitly, we carry with us beliefs about the nature of reality (ontology), about right and wrong (ethics), and about how we come to know the world (epistemology). The doubly challenging thing about these beliefs is they are not only inherently contested, but there is also no worldview-neutral way to determine which ontology, ethic, or epistemology we should adopt. Neither, as I hope to show, is it possible to live our lives—including our lives *as psychologists*—in a worldview-neutral way. Although our discipline emerged in the 19th century with the promise of a method-wrought worldview-neutrality, this promise has not been fulfilled. Indeed, this volume has argued that worldviews are powerfully transmitted through our sociocultural practices such as training (Chapter 2), our psychotherapy (Chapter 3), our research (Chapter 4), and our study of culture (Chapter 5). The remaining question is: what shall we do about this?

This chapter will argue for what may alternatively be called worldview pluralism or worldview diversity. Though the widely used term *viewpoint* diversity[1] is helpful, the notion of *worldview* diversity hopes to expand the contemporary conversation beyond the current focus on political or moral viewpoints, and include the differing ontological and epistemological assumptions that psychologists believe. By employing the notion of *pluralism*, we intend to take advantage of the twofold meaning of the term. The first sense of the term has to do with the simple reality that psychologists are not entirely monolithic in their worldviews. The second sense of the term is aspirational, i.e., the hope that psychology might formally adopt a position that *recognizes and nurtures* the diverse worldviews of its members, employing this diversity to improve science, and providing space to explore the possible connections between those worldviews and psychological thought and practice. The latter half of this chapter offers some initial concepts which we hope will advance the conversation on worldview pluralism within psychology, and, finally, within the viewpoint diversity movement itself. The chapter must begin, however, with an account of the significant obstacles which both impede and necessitate worldview pluralism.

A Certain Blindness in Human Beings—and the Difficulty of Worldview Pluralism

In this account of the obstacles to worldview pluralism, we may start with one of North America's greatest psychologists of belief, William James (1890), who began his treatment of the subject with a common intuition: "everyone knows the difference between imagining a thing and believing in its existence, between supposing a proposition and acquiescing in its truth" (p. 283). In the domain of *worldview* beliefs, it is one thing to "suppose"—either on a conscious or merely intuitive level—ontological, ethical, or epistemological propositions, such as "material reality is all there is," or "psychology should adopt the position of worldview pluralism," or "operational definitions can provide legitimate insight in to psychological phenomena"; it is quite another to *believe* them. How do we know whether we believe them or not? James insisted, quite plausibly, that it's a matter of *feeling*. Belief is "a sort of feeling more allied to the emotions than anything else" (p. 283). Indeed, James refers to "the emotion of belief" (p. 284). When a proposition arouses "the believing reaction" (p. 305), we consciously or intuitively perceive that proposition to be real, or true. Hence, he called belief "the perception of reality" and his account of belief in the *Principles of Psychology* occurs in a chapter by that name. By contrast, when propositions fail to create this feeling, we doubt and perceive such things to be unreal.

This becomes problematic for tolerance and pluralism because people end up living in very different perceptual "worlds" (p. 291), believing or intuiting very different *realities*. Now it is true, James argued, that there are certain realities which *all* human beings seem to believe. The reality of our sensations is one of these things. The reality of our own existence is another. These, however, are scant resources for forging consensus! When it comes to worldviews (part of what James called "belief in objects of theory," p. 311), we can differ radically, and there is no easy intellectual or rational path toward consensus since these beliefs are not primarily derived through cool and rational means. Instead, we tend to believe "those which appeal most urgently to our aesthetic, emotional, and active needs" (p. 312). It isn't that we aren't capable of articulating reasons if called to, it's just that these reasons are likely to be tied to these practical needs.

Worldview pluralism is further complicated by the role of emotion in belief. For James, the more people feel, the more they tend to believe. Though there is fluctuation in the degree to which particular worldview assumptions seem real to us, when we conceive something with fervency, we affirm its existence: "to conceive with passion is *eo ipso* [by that very fact] to affirm" (p. 308). However, and here is the big issue, as Bagehot wrote, passion is often "strongest in those points in which [people] differ most from each other" (p. 308). Our often passionately held worldview beliefs, therefore, are likely to ooze with certainty. To make matters worse, we're by nature inclined to find opposing worldview beliefs unreal, and therefore uninteresting, unworthy, unfathomable, "unbelievable," and perhaps even evil.

In his well-known essay "On a Certain Blindness in Human Beings," James (1899/1958) applied these psychological insights to the problem of pluralism, or of getting along with people whose sense of reality differs radically from our own. This "blindness in human beings," he explained, "is the blindness with which *we all are afflicted* in regard to the feelings of creatures and people different from ourselves" (p. 149, emphasis added). This "ancestral blindness" dulls our sensitivity to the perspective of others. Since, as believers, we all live in different perceptual realities or worlds, we have a tendency to lack empathy or even charity toward those whose values or experiences differ from our own. To illustrate, James tells the story of encountering certain settlements or "coves" in the wilderness of North Carolina which he perceived to be aesthetic atrocities and "unmitigated squalor" (p. 150). But when his Mountaineer guide explained "why, we ain't happy here, unless we are getting one of these coves under cultivation," James wrote, "I instantly felt that I had been losing the whole inward significance of the situation. Because to me the clearing spoke of naught but denudation," he mistakenly believed that "they could tell no other story" (p. 151). That really nails it: our blindness is to the possibility that other stories could be told. And this implies yet another kind of blindness, i.e., to the fact that we ourselves are caught up in our own perceptual world.

Scientific Evidence for This Blindness in Human Beings

Contemporary psychological research bears James out. Long-standing research has illuminated the human tendency to be convinced of the superiority of our own viewpoints. We know, for example, that human beings

have a tendency to resist changing their beliefs even when they are presented with contradictory evidence (belief perseverance); we tend to seek
out information that confirms what were already committed to (confirmation bias). Consistent with both of these classic biases, strong evidence
for "argumentative theory" (Mercier & Sperber, 2011) suggest that human
reason isn't primary oriented toward truth, but rather toward finding support for what we already believe. More recently, emerging support for the
"ideological conflict hypothesis" (Brandt, Reyna, Chambers, Crawford, &
Wetherell, 2014) suggests that prejudicial attitudes are likely not the
domain of *particular* worldviews, but, rather, people generally tend to be
prejudiced against those whom they believe hold opposing worldviews.
There is further evidence that the belief-discrimination link is mediated
by perceived *value violations*, i.e., when we believe that another person's
values violate our own, we're more likely to discriminate (Wetherell, Brandt, &
Reyna, 2013). Indeed, preference for one's own worldview "may stem
from fundamental psychological processes that humans all share" (Brandt
et al., 2014, p. 32). In other words, such worldview-bias and blindness to
the insights of opposing worldview beliefs may be part of human nature,
as James suggested.

The work of Jonathan Haidt has also borne James out. Haidt's work has
provided evidence that our moral reasoning is the "rational tail" of an "intuitive dog" (Haidt, 2012, p. 33ff). When it comes to moral beliefs—which are
a type of worldview belief—intuitions come first and then we often struggle
(and in Haidt's lab, humorously so) to come up with reasons for those intuitions. A few years ago, Haidt (2011)[2] delivered a highly significant conference talk entitled "the bright future of post-partisan social psychology,"
which foregrounded the social element to (moral) worldview beliefs. Moral
commitments, he argues, not only blind us, but they also bind us together.
We tend to assemble into collectives that share a certain set of moral convictions. Among ultra-social species—and unlike other ultra-social species like
bees, wasps, ants, termites, and mole rats—human beings are unique in that
we maintain social solidarity "by circling around sacred objects and principles" which allow 'worshippers' to trust one another. Sacredness, according
to Phil Tetlock, is "any value that a moral community implicitly or explicitly
treats as possessing infinite or transcendental significance." Haidt continues, "when sacred values are threatened, we turn into [what Tetlock calls]
'intuitive theologians,' that is, we use our reasoning not to find the truth,
but to find ways to defend what we hold sacred." He continues: "sacralizing
distorts thinking. These distortions are easy for outsiders to see, but they are
invisible to those inside the force field." So in other words, sacred values,
which all human beings possess, likewise *blind us* to the insights and truths
of those outside of our own communities.

Worldview Blindness in the Discipline of Psychology

Psychology, for all of its insight into the human condition, has at times had difficulty applying its own insights *to itself*. It has, in other words, a "reflexivity" problem. We quite readily and correctly affirm that *individuals* suffer from a certain blindness, cognitive biases, and emotional thinking. But psychologists, we imply, have risen above the human condition. This is where Haidt's talk becomes historic, and particularly relevant to our discussion: "But moral force fields are not only found in religious communities. They can operate in academic fields as well." Haidt (2011) shows that social psychology is dominated by a particular set of ethical assumptions which not only bind the discipline together but also blind the discipline to certain possible types of explanations. In a dramatic demonstration on the floor of the annual meeting of the Society for Personality and Social Psychology, the vast majority of attendees indicated they were politically liberal and a fraction of 1 percent confessed to being conservative. After Haidt's talk, there has been an ever-growing awareness of ideological (or *worldview*) homogeneity in psychology. In a recent issue of *Behavioral and Brain Sciences*, for example, Duarte, Crawford, Stern, Haidt, Jussim, and Tetlock (2015) write a target essay providing further empirical evidence of a particular bias within social psychology. In 1996, liberals outnumbered conservatives in psychology by a ratio of 4:1. By 2012, the imbalance had grown to 14:1. A follow-up to this review (Haidt & Jussim, 2016) has provided more evidence of this striking imbalance.

It's too easy to get distracted by the political labels "liberal" and "conservative" here. What's crucial and at stake is that Duarte et al. (2015) *are dealing with worldview assumptions*, particularly moral assumptions. For some, the moral imperative to fight for justice for the oppressed is paramount. For others, the moral imperative of personal responsibility is paramount. These insights complement one of the basic theses of this volume, that psychology has certain privileged worldview beliefs, whether they be individualism, naturalism, or, in this case, moral/political beliefs. The point is that the discipline has given preference to one set of worldview beliefs and been "blind" (in a Jamesian sense) to the insights of alternative assumptions. This too, and perhaps especially, makes worldview pluralism in psychology a profound challenge.

The Deep Roots of Worldview Blindness in the History of the North American University

Worldview pluralism would seem to have two strikes against it, then. As James and psychological science attest, worldview blindness is a powerful part of human psychology—that's strike one. As Haidt and others recite the statistics within psychology of a powerful allegiance to a single set of moral worldview commitments, alongside the evidence in this volume for other worldview biases in the discipline, the possibility of worldview pluralism seems even less plausible—that's strike two. But there's yet another factor which would seem to make worldview pluralism within psychology even less likely, and that's the historical context in which this issue emerges. In short, worldview blindness has dominated North American psychology for about 250 years, so the possibility of reform would seem bleak indeed.

Following historian George Marsden (1994), it may be argued that a crucial change in North American higher education began during the middle of the 18th century. Prior to that point, during what we may call the confessional era[3] (1636–1758) of psychological thought, colleges tended to be sectarian schools where worldview commitments were stated clearly and explicitly. There was no pretended neutrality—faculty were expected to believe the orthodoxy of the academy and uphold it in their teaching. The main psychologies of this era were contained in theological textbooks, such as William Ames's (1643/1968) *Marrow of Theology*. As the colonial religious landscape became more diverse, however, it became difficult to maintain narrowly defined theological orthodoxies while simultaneously remaining truly public institutions. Typically, colleges chose the route of public engagement and broad appeal rather than disengagement and sectarianism (Marsden, 1994).

In order to maintain their status as public institutions, however, these colleges did not embrace confessional or worldview pluralism—where a multitude of different creeds could be recognized—rather, the "non-sectarian" solution they adopted was to employ the "neutral" methods of the Scottish Enlightenment. The psychology of the day would be based upon the objective observation "of" facts of consciousness," which would then be inductively arranged (via the method of the revered Francis Bacon) into systems of moral and mental philosophy, the proto-psychology of the 18th and 19th centuries (Fuchs, 2000). When these proto-psychologies are studied in the 21st century, however, it is clear they were far from worldview-neutral. For example, Brown University president Francis Wayland's (1837/1963) best-selling moral philosophy textbook articulated a "doctrine of general consequences" (p. 110) where harmful outcomes were taken as evidence that certain behaviors were outside of God's will. Not exactly the kind of conclusion psychologists would tend to draw today! Clearly, then, supposedly neutral methods were being used in a hegemonically Christian educational context in which, lo and behold, all the data clearly pointed to the truth of Christianity![4]

Psychological thought in North America has gone through at least two worldview shifts since then. During what we might call a "transitional era"

from approximately 1879 to 1913, there was a movement away from traditional Protestant worldview to a "liberal Protestant" worldview, which
emphasized traditional morality but rejected dogma, embracing instead a
non-materialist, evolutionary outlook (White, 2008). This revolution (Smith,
2003) was likewise carried out under the guise of methodological purity—
the "New Psychology," it was repeated again and again, was primarily about
becoming a *real* science, embracing the new scientific methods of Wundt
and others. But the findings of this new psychology were understood to
uphold the beliefs of liberal Protestantism (Pickren, 2000). Indeed, William
James's classic *Principles of Psychology* is filled with moral exhortations
consistent with this era.

What we might call the "secular era" of psychology began arguably with
John Watson's (1913) "Behaviorist Manifesto." Once again, there was a
call for methodological purity, an emphasis on behavior and a movement
away from introspection. But a new worldview was being smuggled in, as
Watson proclaimed that there was "no dividing line between man and brute"
(p. 158), behaviorism would come to believe that animal research would suffice in the quest to understand human behavior. Though, of course, psychology no longer abides by the methodological rigors of radical behaviorism,
its implicit commitment to naturalism (and relegation of other ontologies)
remains (as Chapter 4 argues).

This rough outline of North American psychology's history suggests that
several highly significant worldview changes have taken place over the
last few centuries, but these shifts were never above board. Instead, each
era cloaked its significant worldview change under the guise of methodological purity. Also, a general pattern of interpretation emerged where the
agreed-upon data of the psychological science[5] of the era were understood to
un-problematically support the regnant worldview. The circularity of these
arguments was (and still is) lost on all but those who did (or do) not share
the dominant worldview.

Are There Alternatives to Worldview Blindness in Psychology? The Possibility of Coexistence

This historical narrative suggests the existence of massive historical forces
that could very well be strike three for worldview pluralism. Discrimination
against the worldviews of outgroups appears to be deeply woven into human
nature, into the discipline itself, and obscured by dissonance-reducing institutional structures which allow us to continue with a clean conscience that
at least *we* are open-minded and scientific, all the while perpetuating worldview blindness. But we mustn't give up so easily—the integrity of our discipline is at stake.

As legal scholar John Inazu (2016) points out in his book *Confident Pluralism*, we really have three options when it comes to dealing with what "John Rawls called. . .'the fact of pluralism'—'the recognition that we live in [an academic discipline] of 'a plurality of conflicting, and indeed incommensurable, conceptions of meaning, value and purpose of human life.'" (pp. 4–5). The worldview blindness of psychology is a form of "control," one of Inazu's (2015) three options. Control occurs when we "feign agreement by ignoring or minimizing our stark differences" (p. 128) Unstated but dominant worldview assumptions are like the proverbial water in which the fish swim, taken for granted by all except those poor creatures who lack gills. "We hold conferences," he writes, which seem to be "expressing unity and solidarity" (p. 128) when in reality dissenting voices or opinions are unexpressed. Clearly, control is not the ideal solution to the fact of pluralism.

Another possibility is chaos. We see this in the political situation in the United States, where the expression of diverse opinions is often hateful. James (1899/1958), describing the "unhealthy and regrettable" political situation of his day, captures ours perfectly:

> The unhealthiness consists solely in the fact that one-half of our fellow-countrymen remain entirely blind to the internal significance of the lives of the other half. They miss the joys and sorrows, they fail to feel the moral virtue, and they do not guess the presence of the intellectual ideals.
>
> (p. 189)

It is this unwillingness to empathize with the other, to see the virtue and struggles of those with whom we disagree that leads to a chaotic shouting match. And opponents of worldview pluralism within psychology may likewise fear that such openness could lead to a "confusion of tongues" in our discipline, distraction by irrelevancies at best, inanities at worst. To these, I ask that they hear us out.

The third and best way of dealing with the fact of pluralism, and the best alternative to worldview blindness is what Inazu (2015) calls "confident pluralism." He writes:

> There is another possibility that better embraces the reality of our deepest differences: confident pluralism. Confident pluralism insists that. . .our shared existence is not only possible, but necessary. Instead of the elusive goal of *E pluribus unum* ("Out of many, one"), confident pluralism suggests a more modest possibility—that we can live together in our "many-ness." It does not require Pollyanna-ish illusions that we will resolve our differences and live happily ever after.

Instead, it asks us to pursue a common existence in spite of our deeply held differences.

(p. 128)

Coexistence is a better approach for our discipline. It's where psychologists are allowed to be themselves, to come out of their respective worldview closets, and to openly explore the connections between their psychologies and their deepest convictions.

Some of Inazu's critics do not emphasize the logic of his argumentation, but rather his optimism. They fear that society is simply too divided to behave in such a civil and open-minded way. Given the acrimonious nature of public discourse, his critics may well be right. But there is good reason to be optimistic about psychology, despite all of the significant obstacles. Not only has our understanding of worldview bias increased as the foregoing attests, but, I hope to show, there may be sufficient resources and agreement within our discipline to make progress on worldview pluralism.

How Can We Coexist in Psychology? Moving Toward Worldview Awareness in Psychology

If successful, this concluding chapter has taken us some distance toward the first step toward worldview pluralism in psychology, i.e., recognizing our propensity toward worldview blindness, which is the tendency to take our worldview convictions as *given*, in need of no explanation, as an accurate perception of reality, so much so that we may not even realize we have such assumptions. Further, worldview blindness is the tendency to be prejudiced against those viewpoints which oppose our own, to take opposing viewpoints as unreal or perhaps even evil. In short, the preceding considerations suggest that our certainty about our worldview beliefs is more likely due to the fact that we are human than to the fact that we are right.

The opposite of worldview blindness is worldview awareness. It is the process of making the implicit explicit, and becoming aware of the worldviews that are actually in play—in ourselves, in our opponents, and in the academic discipline we serve. Thankfully, we live in a time of growing worldview awareness as the moral/political biases of the academy have been made explicit by the "viewpoint diversity" movement (heterodoxacademy.org). This volume has aimed to take an additional step, by highlighting other worldview beliefs that prevail in psychology.

It should be noted that both the viewpoint diversity movement and the preceding chapters have focused on what we might call *contested* worldview assumptions, i.e., those worldview beliefs in which psychologists *differ* from one another. Still, it has been widely recognized that pluralism requires more than recognition of difference—after all, if we have absolutely nothing in common, our prospects of coexistence are bleak indeed. Inazu's analysis, as we will see, suggests that there can be some areas of agreement that form the basis of confident pluralism. We might say, then, that while contested worldview beliefs *necessitate* worldview pluralism, it is our consensual worldview beliefs that *make worldview pluralism possible.* So, part of worldview awareness within psychology includes an understanding of consensual worldview assumptions.

To make sense of the following, it's important to make explicit a distinction that has heretofore only been implicit, i.e., that between one's "worldview" (WV) or the entire constellation of one's ontological, ethical, and epistemological beliefs, and "individual worldview beliefs" (IWBs), i.e., particular beliefs about ontological, ethical, and epistemological issues. It's clear that people from very different worldviews (WVs) can share individual worldview beliefs (IWBs). For example, many naturalists and theists can agree in the existence of the mind (an ontological belief), even though their understanding of the mind may vary greatly. Many liberals and conservatives can agree that poverty is bad (an ethical belief), though they may have very different understandings of its causes and cures. So the attempt to find consensual worldview beliefs is a quest to find consensual IWBs, not an attempt to find consensual WVs.

This chapter will explore the possibility of finding consensual IWBs in two ways. First, we'll look at what we believe to be consensual *ethical and political* worldview assumptions of most psychologists, regardless of theoretical orientation. Given the enormous emphasis today on the ethical/political beliefs that divide psychologists, it may come as some shock that psychologists may very well agree on some bedrock principles. Acknowledging and re-committing to agreed-upon assumptions should set the stage for worldview pluralism within the field more broadly. Second, we'll turn our attention to the viewpoint diversity movement itself, and the sticky question whether worldview pluralism is possible in mainstream psychological science, a discipline that was, as Chapter 4 and this chapter have argued, born of the WV of naturalism.

The Shared Ethical Assumptions of Psychologists

In some sense, identifying the consensual ethical assumptions of psychologists should be rather straightforward. All research in North America must pass muster through Institutional Review Boards (IRBs in the States) or Research Ethics Boards (REBs in Canada) which are governed by very similar ethical codes. Membership in the APA requires that members promise to uphold the association's *Ethical Principles of Psychologists and Code of Conduct.* Likewise, members of the Canadian

Psychological Association abide by the *Canadian Code of Ethics for Psychologists*. But there are potentially other consensual ethical assumptions uniting psychologists which would facilitate worldview pluralism in particular. Here we return to the work of John Inazu.

Inazu argues that a common existence is possible through civil practice or virtues, which we can re-frame as a matter of ethical worldview commitments. Inazu (2015) explains, "if enough of us embrace these aspirations, we may be able to sustain a consensus for confident pluralism, even as we draw from eclectic and blended antecedents" (p. 131). In other words, we may have significant disagreements at the level of entire worldviews, we may still nevertheless agree on several individual virtues/ethical standards.

The first of these is tolerance, "the most important aspiration of confident pluralism" (Inazu, 2015, p. 132). Our worldview disagreements may run deep indeed, and we may find the positions of others reprehensible. "As the philosopher Bernard Williams has observed, tolerance is most needed when people find others' beliefs or practices 'deeply unacceptable' or 'blasphemously, disastrously, obscenely wrong.' The basic difficulty of tolerance, Williams notes, is that we need it 'only for the intolerable'" (p. 132). Etymologically the word "tolerance" includes a root that means "endurance" (Inazu, 2016, p. 87). So tolerance is in no way an endorsing of the other's viewpoint.

The next virtue is humility. If tolerance is the most important aspiration, humility "requires even greater self-reflection and self-discipline than tolerance" (Inazu, 2015, p. 132). We've briefly explored why this is the case—our minds are prone to overconfidence in the correctness of our own opinions and in the incorrectness of our opponents'. Inazu, not a psychologist, addresses this perfectly when he says, "our human faculties are inherently limited—our ability to think, reason, and reflect is less than perfect, a limitation that leaves open the possibility that we can be wrong." Further, one of the main characteristics of worldview beliefs is that they are unprovable, and this, too, is grounds for humility. Inazu says:

> This kind of humility is based on the limits of what we can prove, not on claims about what is true. For this reason, it should not be mistaken for relativism. Humility leaves open the possibility that there is right and wrong and good and evil. Humility does not impugn our confidence in truth, but it calls for a recognition that our beliefs often stem from contested premises that others do not share.
>
> (p. 132)

Psychologists—of all people—should understand this. As James (1899/1958) wrote, "cannot we at least use our sense of our own blindness to make us more cautious?" (p. 172).

Finally, Inazu recommends patience. If nothing else, worldview beliefs are characterized by confidence, as we have seen. Haidt (2012) says we have "righteous minds" not merely "moral minds" because we tend to be judgmental and convinced of our own righteousness (p. xix). But our opponents are likewise confident in their beliefs (and perhaps righteousness). So persuasion cannot be our first aim as we embrace worldview pluralism. But we will of course attempt to present our own sides of the story as best we can. Perhaps we'll win some. But, as Inazu says, "dialogue and persuasion usually take time." Inazu (2015) notes:

> Many of us will need patience to get to know one another across our differences, to stumble toward dialogue across the awkward distance that separates us. Sometimes we will need patience to endure differences that will not be overcome. Patience also encourages efforts to listen, understand, and perhaps even to empathize. Those activities are not the same as accepting or embracing another view. It may turn out that patience leads us to a deeper realization of the evil or depravity of an opposing belief. But we can at least assume a posture that moves beyond caricatured dismissals of others before we even hear what they have to say.
>
> (p. 133)

Again, psychologists should recognize this. Our "certain blindness" is part of the human condition and, as James (1899/1958) wrote, "it is vain to hope for this state of things to alter much" (p. 171). We will need patience indeed.

To these virtues, I would add two. The first comes from what William James (1899/1958) called "sympathy" (p. 176) or even "reverence, and love" (p. 188). There needs to be a willingness to understand, a desire to perceive the joy of the other person ("to miss the joy is to miss all" (p. 152); James thought this line from Robert Lewis Stephenson was key). As Carl Rogers (1980) put it, people need to feel "prized" (p. 116). Instead of dismissing or squashing the central values of our fellow psychologists, we ought to yearn to know one another better. Inazu's values tend to emphasize unpleasant aspects of worldview pluralism, endurance and long-suffering. But Jamesian sympathy is a striving for a genuine delight in the other whenever possible.

Finally, I would add to this courage. As we open up our hearts to the viewpoints of other psychologists, as we come to see the joy that they possess, we may be struck by the fact that they enjoy a more compelling vision than we do. And this would suggest the need to revise our own worldview commitments. Because our worldviews are among the most precious things we possess, it takes tremendous courage to be willing to risk these as we enter into genuine dialogue among fellow psychologists. To be so open to other opinions is risky. If we're truly open-minded, we may find ourselves *persuaded*.

There is another, equally important, side to courage, i.e., the courage to speak up. Although members of suppressed worldview communities within psychology may for understandable reasons be accustomed to keeping their opinions to themselves, genuine worldview pluralism is hindered to the extent that psychologists are afraid to "come out" and share their actual experiences and convictions. We should encourage one another to be to more transparent, particularly by being more tolerant, humble, patient, sympathetic, and courageous ourselves.

Worldview Pluralism as a Shared Democratic Ideal

North American psychologists work within the context of democratic governments and might share a common commitment to democratic ideals (perhaps even going as far as James (1899/1958), who referred to "the religion of democracy," p. 178). Could this common commitment also provide consensual IWBs that might further advance worldview pluralism within psychology?

The possibility of democratic grounds for worldview pluralism has been recognized at least to some extent within the North American university, the best example of which might be the emergence of aboriginal studies within Canada. The Truth and Reconciliation Commission of Canada (2015) has taken significant steps toward recognizing the long and horrific history of oppression of aboriginal people, particularly the century-long "cultural genocide" (p. 1) of residential schools in which aboriginal children would be forcibly removed from their "savage" parents to teach them—as the first Prime Minister of Canada put it—"to acquire the habits and modes of thought of white men" (p. 2). In view of the Commission's work, there is a nationwide effort to make Canada "a more prosperous, just, and inclusive democracy" (p. 7). Part of this work ensures that authentic aboriginal voices have their own place within publically funded research universities. In line with this, the Social Sciences and Humanities Research Council (SSHRC)—the major federal funding agency for psychology and other social sciences in Canada—supports "aboriginal research," and their (2016) published guidelines to evaluate applications for public funding recognize as legitimate "research incorporating Aboriginal knowledge systems (including ontologies, epistemologies and methodologies)." Here's the point: no one claims that aboriginal studies have a place within the public university because the worldviews of indigenous peoples are universally recognized as true or are a new orthodoxy of the academy. Rather, one animating idea is that the indigenous people of Canada have their own cultures and worldviews that—*on democratic grounds*—need to be respected, heard, and nurtured.

It would seem that other worldviews—particularly those that already exist within the discipline but have been suppressed—should likewise be respected, heard, and nurtured in psychology. Granted, the use of democratic ideals within the university may raise concerns about the creation of an undesirable situation in which the most zany or evil ideals are legitimized. But the greater risk, I would argue, is the perpetuation of worldview blindness—particularly that of the dominant/majority ingroup—which is inclined to label outgroup worldviews as zany and evil in the first place. The only requirement for inclusion ought to be a willingness to embrace the consensual disciplinary values of tolerance, humility, patience, sympathy, and courage. If all worldview groups within psychology—majority and minority—can sincerely embrace these five ideals, we have nothing to fear and much to gain. Indeed, the benefits would go well beyond democratic fairness, as the section on viewpoint diversity below suggests.

With these preliminary thoughts in mind, we may turn to a discussion of consensual democratic IWBs that might structure our lives within psychology. John Inazu's (2016) *Confident Pluralism* is helpful here once again. In addition to—and in some way flowing out of (p. 10)—the shared civic virtues of tolerance, humility, and patience, Inazu (working in an American context) argues that a confident pluralism can also be understood as having a basis in Constitutional law. The US Constitution is a foundational statement of democratic principles, and has influenced many other democracies in the western world, so the principles he articulates might have wide application. Specifically, Inazu's argument provides a useful democratic framework for thinking about how a worldview-plural psychology might organize itself.

Inazu's democratic/constitutional line of argumentation has three main "prongs." The first prong, *the right of association*, is "the most important constitutional commitment of confident pluralism" (Inazu, 2015, p. 129) and could be interpreted in two possible ways for psychology, one, ironically, in a way that suppresses worldview diversity and another in a way that encourages it. Inazu explains that "part of the right of association entails discrimination—a meaningful right of association will permit voluntary groups to exclude." As an example, he talks about Wellesley College, which "discriminates against men and unexceptionally performing high school students." Likewise, "the Mormon Tabernacle Choir discriminates against non-Mormons and bad singers." Continuing, he explains that "within the voluntary groups of civil society, we tolerate forms of discrimination that would elsewhere be impermissible" (p. 130).

There are two possible ways this could be applied in the discipline of psychology. One way would be to conceive of psychologists as one ideologically homogeneous voluntary group. The discipline could take the recent evidence of liberal bias in psychology, for example, and suggest that this is now going to be the orthodoxy of the discipline, and discriminate against those who do not share this orthodoxy. Although there is evidence that such discrimination takes place already (Duarte et al., 2015), it seems highly unlikely that psychology would want to take such an extreme and prejudicial approach that would *mandate* that all worldview minorities leave the discipline.

The other, worldview-plural way that this could be applied in psychology is to think of "voluntary groups" *within* psychology. That is, members of various worldview communities should be allowed the right of association within the field of psychology. Within APA or CPA, for example, there ought to be divisions (APA) or sections (CPA) for all worldview communities already within the field that desire a place where they can talk and work together. Such divisions and sections already exist for some worldview communities, particularly those consistent with the current worldview biases of the discipline. Worldview pluralism in psychology would insist that *all* worldview groups within psychology have the right of association, not only those who share the dominant value system. The entire discipline would benefit, as I hope to show. By contrast, one way to perpetuate worldview blindness and control is to prevent non-dominant worldview groups within psychology from talking to each other.

Inazu's (2015) second constitutional prong of for pluralism is *public forums*, or:

> physical and virtual spaces where citizens come together to voice their dissent, opposition, and discontent. Public forums can be actual places, such as town halls, but they can also be non-physical or virtual spaces. Public colleges and universities create public forums when they allow students to form their own organizations; local governments often create public forums when they solicit comments on a website.
>
> (p. 130)

Applying this idea to psychology, worldview pluralism would, then, affirm that psychology as a discipline, its conferences and journals, ought to be conceived of as a "public forum" in which members of the guild can—in mutually agreeable and helpful ways—"come together to voice their dissent, opposition, and discontent."

Inazu (2015) points to a deficiency in current practice in which "political protestors in public forums are often relegated to physically distant and ironically named 'free-speech zones'" (p. 130). This is a reminder that creating special divisions in the APA or sections in the CPA for various worldview groups would not go far enough if these become ironic "free-speech zones" while in the public forums they must remain closeted as they have always been. On the other hand, if we viewed such divisions as providing the right of association for like-minded individuals, and the discipline itself as a public forum in which the fruit of these "sectarian" discussions can be shared with the broader community for the common good, this might help us all overcome our native blindness to our own perspectives and to each other's insights.

Inazu's third and final democratic prong for pluralism is *public funding*: "Finally, it is important that we preserve access to generally available public funding, regardless of ideology" (p. 131). He makes very interesting point that tax-exempt status applies to very different groups, "The pro-choice group and the pro-life group, religious groups of all stripes (or no stripe), hunting organizations and animal-rights groups—the federal tax deduction benefits them all" (p. 131). When one side calls for the other to be stripped of its tax exemption, we've lost sight of the pluralistic ideal. Likewise, in the discipline of psychology, research and scholarship funding should not be limited to preferred worldview groups, but there should be a concerted effort to distribute funding to all, especially marginalized worldview groups—the example of SSHRC's funding of aboriginal research in Canada is an excellent example of this. Such a step would ensure that each worldview community can develop its own psychological thinking so that it can be presented, as Mill put it, in its "most plausible and persuasive form" (Jussim, Haidt, & Martin, n.d.)

Is the "Viewpoint Diversity" Movement an Example of Worldview Pluralism?

The viewpoint diversity movement has been mentioned several times in this chapter, and it has been suggested that there is some connection between it and the worldview pluralism advocated herein. It's therefore fitting to explore in a bit more detail the compatibility between its vision and ours. Again, the viewpoint diversity movement (heterodoxacademy.org), within psychology and beyond, begins with the recognition of a particular kind of worldview bias within the mainstream university, discusses how this bias diminishes science, and calls for a diversity of viewpoints (particularly moral/political viewpoints) to improve science. I shall elaborate on this a bit below.

The crucial preliminary point, however, is that—within psychology—"viewpoint diversity" is a movement within mainstream psychological science (MPS). So we need to ask whether worldview pluralism is possible within MPS before we can ask if the viewpoint diversity movement is compatible with worldview pluralism. By MPS I refer to the quantitatively oriented discipline emphasized in most undergraduate and graduate education, exemplified by professional organizations like the Association for Psychological Science (APS) and their journals, and what's taken for granted when most psychologists today refer to the term "psychological science." If any psychology could claim to have the ability to pursue truth while transcending the influence of worldview—and, by consequence, the claims of worldview diversity—it would seem to be MPS. In what follows, however, I hope to make a few paradoxical points about MPS. On the one hand, I hope to show that MPS is not worldview-neutral at all, but rather is based upon a number of ontological and epistemological assumptions that not all psychologists hold. On the other hand, despite—and, indeed, *because of*—this non-neutrality vis-à-vis *certain* worldview assumptions, a truncated form of worldview pluralism is nevertheless possible within MPS.

How can MPS be non-neutral and yet worldview-plural? Isn't this a contradiction? My personal sense is that MPS brings together researchers from diverse WVs (in the sense of interconnected systems of worldview beliefs) because these researchers share a set of individual worldview beliefs (IWBs, as discussed above) that make MPS possible. Many psychologists outside of MPS reject these IWBs (such as *some* qualitative researchers), yet, within MPS these shared assumptions enable an otherwise-worldview-diverse community to work together. Let's begin, then, by discussing some of these IWBs.

Ontologically, the MPS community tends to assume that minds exist; that there are causal connections between mind, behavior, and environment; that the mind is connected to biology, including genes and brain; that psychological and behavioral phenomena have a certain lawfulness (even if that lawfulness is merely probabilistic and aggregate-level only). Further, the community assumes the capacity of the human mind to understand this lawfulness. Without such assumptions the current research practices of MPS would make very little sense.

Although these assumptions may seem to be expressions of the worldview of naturalism, it turns out that these assumptions are embraced by members of different worldview communities. Certainly, the methods of MPS were born under the influence of the worldview of naturalism (Chapter 4 and this chapter), but many researchers within the MPS community do not embrace metaphysical naturalism. The most obvious example I know of this would be the existence of psychology departments (such as my own) within the 115 member campuses of the evangelical Council of Christian Colleges and Universities (cccu.org). These departments overwhelmingly teach the methods and subfields of MPS, yet are populated by theists. To counter the claim that these theists are simply unknowingly presupposing naturalism, philosopher Alvin Plantinga (2011) argues paradoxically that ontological assumptions such as these cohere with theism, not naturalism! But the point here is not to argue whose WVs better cohere with the shared IWBs of MPS. It's just to show that folks from different WVs find a place for these assumptions. This serves to support the general point—that MPS is non-neutral ontologically, but these shared IWBs make it possible for psychologists with different worldviews (WVs) to participate in MPS.

Epistemologically, the MPS community tends to presuppose a number of ideas. For example, that it is possible to create measures that imperfectly but usefully translate bio-psycho-social reality into numbers; that learning about the association between measures in samples, whether through correlation, regression, or other multivariate techniques, can provide useful insight into a wide range of phenomena; that learning about mean differences between groups in experimental or quasi-experimental designs provides important information concerning a whole range of factors that influence psychological and behavioral reality; that inferences from samples to populations depend on other assumptions, such as the legitimacy of imagining hypothetical populations whose scores on variables are normally distributed, or that tentative conclusions about data may be drawn by comparing an observed result with a hypothetical comparison distribution assuming that "the null hypothesis" is true, i.e., that there was no effect.

It should be noted that these consensual epistemological assumptions are continually being revised. Within a decade we may no longer be assuming the variables are normally distributed or that estimating the probability of observing a particular outcome given the null hypothesis is a legitimate way to go. There are, of course, significant methodological reforms going on in psychology at this very moment, and these amount to a negotiation regarding what the MPS community will assume epistemologically.

Once again, researchers in MPS holding diverse worldviews seem to have found a place for these epistemological IWBs. Though naturalistically inclined scientists may argue—in a manner analogous to the positivists of old—that psychological knowledge is possible *only* through empirical methods such as these; others might hold that tradition, literature, philosophy, revelation, or other sources also provide valid psychological insight (albeit insights that cannot be merely asserted within MPS). Certainly, this is the case for the aforementioned psychologists within the CCCU. Likewise, the viewpoint diversity movement has put a spotlight on examples of viewpoint minorities (e.g., libertarians) participating in MPS, showing that those with different worldviews have already found a place for these IWBs.

MPS, then, far from a completely worldview-neutral endeavor, is full of individual worldview beliefs (IWBs) that are held in common by people from diverse worldviews. By presupposing these IWBs, psychologists with diverse worldviews are able to work side by side in their common pursuit of psychological knowledge. With this background in place, we may finally address the question: is worldview pluralism possible *within MPS*? I think the answer to this question is a qualified yes. Obviously, insofar as the methods of MPS presuppose IWBs such as those discussed above, it is not ontologically or epistemologically "neutral," so any worldview pluralism within MPS must of necessity be a truncated or limited variety, i.e., a world-view pluralism for psychologists who find a place for the consensual IWBs of MPS within their entire network of worldview beliefs (but not for those psychologists who reject these IWBs). However, if psychological scientists agree to presuppose *only* these consensual IWBs, and diligently guard against presupposing or smuggling in *contested* worldview assumptions, a limited form of worldview pluralism should be possible within MPS.

This is precisely what has begun to happen in the viewpoint diversity movement, which has taken the first steps in the direction of a *worldview-plural psychological science*—a very exciting development indeed. Again, the focus of this community of researchers has been on how one set of (left-leaning) moral/political values has come to dominate MPS, creating a need for more political diversity within the field to ensure "institutionalized disconfirmation," so that researchers don't get sloppy and allow a discipline-wide confirmation bias to take hold. Although it's never explicitly stated, what's happening in the viewpoint diversity movement, in other words, is a community of researchers which shares one set of viewpoints (the shared ontological and epistemological IWBs of MPS) is bringing attention to how non-shared moral/political worldview beliefs are being privileged within the discipline, to the detriment of MPS. For example, Duarte et al. (2015) show how the dominant and unchecked ethical/political worldview beliefs of the mainstream have diminished the quality of social psychology research by creeping into the methods and paradigms of social psychology, by becoming embedded within operational definitions themselves, by limiting the sorts of research questions and programs available, and even by perpetuating negative but inaccurate stereotypes toward worldview outgroups. They argue that a more ideologically diverse MPS would be much more likely to identify and correct such bias, increasing the likelihood of generating "broadly valid and generalizable conclusions" (p. 7).

Although this volume strongly implies that the viewpoint diversity movement within MPS needs to include other, non-political worldview beliefs, this movement toward a worldview-plural psychological science is nevertheless very encouraging and finds an important place within the worldview pluralism that we advocate in this book. But it is crucial to remember that psychology is broader than MPS, and some psychologists—including several authors in this volume—reject the IWBs of MPS. It is crucial to remember this because MPS—as the purveyor of the dominant epistemology of the discipline—has been one of the biggest perpetuators of worldview blindness within psychology. We see this blindness when psychological scientists presume that *theirs* is the Only True Epistemology and that other psychologies aren't real psychologies or have nothing to offer MPS.

So one of the great goals of worldview pluralism would be a more reflexive, worldview-aware MPS which recognizes its non-neutrality vis-à-vis worldviews, its corresponding limitations and blind spots, and, crucially, its need for other non-MPS psychologies to flourish. A true worldview pluralism would sanction the development of alternative psychologies that reflect the diverse worldviews of psychologists, including psychologies which reject the IWBs of MPS. It would—along the lines Haidt has suggested— engage in some affirmative action, trying to bring in under-represented worldview communities (in Canada, many psychology departments are hiring aboriginal psychologists, for example). In allowing a thousand flowers to bloom, MPS would benefit, too. Indeed, a case can be made that the viewpoint diversity movement *needs* worldview pluralism as described in this chapter, and here's why: As Haidt and others emphasize, in order for viewpoint diversity within MPS to bear fruit, minority opinions must be expressed *in their most refined form*. One of their favorite quotes from John Stewart Mill's *On Liberty*:

> He who knows only his own side of the case knows little of that. His reasons may be good, and no one may have been able to refute them. But if he is equally unable to refute the reasons on the opposite side, if he does not so much as know what they are, he has no ground for preferring either opinion . . . Nor is it enough that he should hear the opinions of adversaries from his own teachers, presented as they state them, and accompanied by what they offer as refutations. He must be able to hear them from persons who actually believe them . . . he must know them in their most plausible and persuasive form.
>
> (as quoted by Jussim et al., n.d.)

But how, precisely, will worldview minority opinions and psychologies come to be expressed "in their most plausible and persuasive form" if the entire discipline—including the training opportunities afforded to such minorities (Chapter 2)—is biased against those very opinions? Simply hiring a few token representatives of those opinions is not enough because such hires will not have experienced the proper conditions in which such articulations are possible. It's only when different worldview communities are treated in accord with the ethical and democratic values expressed above that these conditions will be possible. And all boats will rise.

***

As the historical narrative outlined in the beginning of this chapter attests, worldview pluralism has been a long time coming in the North American university; we've gone from one dominant worldview to the next. But we have hope that psychology—and the university more generally—may be entering into a new, pluralistic era in which our understanding of our tendency toward worldview blindness, our recognition of certain key shared ethical and democratic values, and our shared yearning to better understand the human condition, are leading to a broader, more inclusive, and ultimately more satisfying discipline of psychology.

Notes

1 See heterodoxacademy.org
2 Quotes from this talk are taken from an online version of the same: https://vimeo.com/19822295
3 In what follows, I summarize the worldview-sensitive narrative I've been developing in my history of psychology course.
4 We see the same thing in Yale President Noah Porter's (1884) moral philosophy textbook in which the psychological data provide evidence of Christianity.
5 It's important to remember that prior to the New Psychology, the proto-psychology of the early- and mid-nineteenth century claimed scientific status for itself, as evidenced by titles such as "intellectual science," and "moral science."

References

Ames, W. (1643/1968). *The marrow of theology* (J. D. Eusden, Trans.). Grand Rapids, MI: Baker Books.

Brandt, M. J., Reyna, C., Chambers, J. R., Crawford, J. T., & Wetherell, G. (2014). The ideological-conflict hypothesis: Intolerance among both liberals and conservatives. *Current Directions in Psychological Science, 23*, 27–34.

Duarte, J. L., Crawford, J. T., Stern, C., Haidt, J., Jussim, L., & Tetlock, P. E. (2015). Political diversity will improve social psychological science. *Behavioral and Brain Sciences, 38*, 1–58.

Fuchs, A. H. (2000). Contributions of American mental philosophers to psychology in the United States. *History of Psychology, 3*, 3–19.

Haidt, J. (2011). *The bright future of post-partisan social psychology*. Paper presented at the annual meeting of the Society for Personality and Social Psychology, San Antonio, TX.

Haidt, J. (2012). *The righteous mind: Why good people are divided by politics and religion*. New York: Vintage.

Haidt, J., & Jussim, L. (2016, February). Psychological science and viewpoint diversity. *Observer, 29*, 5–7.

Inazu, J. (2015). Across the great divides: Why America needs a more confident pluralism. *The Hedgehog Review, 17*, 126–137.

Inazu, J. (2016). *Confident pluralism: Surviving and thriving through deep difference*. Chicago, IL: University of Chicago Press.

James, W. (1890). *The principles of psychology* (Vol. II). New York: H. Holt and Company.

James, W. (1899/1958). *Talks to teachers.* New York: Norton.

Jussim, L., Haidt, J., & Martin, C. (n.d.). *The problem.* Retrieved from http://heterodoxacademy.org/problems/

Marsden, G. M. (1994). *The soul of the American university: From Protestant establishment to established nonbelief.* New York: Oxford University Press.

Mercier, H., & Sperber, D. (2011). Why do humans reason? Arguments for an argumentative theory. *Behavioral and Brain Sciences, 34,* 57–111.

Pickren, W. (2000). A whisper of salvation: American psychologists and religion in the popular press, 1884–1908. *American Psychologist, 55,* 1022–1024.

Plantinga, A. (2011). *Where the conflict really lies: Science, religion, and naturalism.* New York: Oxford University Press.

Porter, N. (1884). *The elements of moral science.* New York: Charles Scribner's Sons.

Rogers, C. R. (1980). *A way of being.* Boston: Houghton Mifflin.

Smith, C. (Ed.). (2003). *The secular revolution: Power, interests, and conflict in the secularization of American public life.* Berkeley: University of California Press.

Social Sciences and Humanities Research Council of Canada. (2016, June). *Guidelines for the merit review of aboriginal research.* Retrieved from www.sshrc-crsh.gc.ca/funding-financement/merit_review-evaluation_du_merite/guidelines_research-lignes_directrices_recherche-eng.aspx

Truth and Reconciliation Commission of Canada. (2015). *Honouring the truth, reconciling for the future: Summary of the final report of the Truth and Reconciliation Commission of Canada.* Retrieved from www.trc.ca

Watson, J. B. (1913). Psychology as the behaviorist views it. *Psychological Review, 20,* 158–177.

Wayland, F. (1837/1963). *The elements of moral science* (J. L. Blau Ed.). Cambridge, MA: Belknap.

Wetherell, G., Brandt, M. J., & Reyna, C. (2013). Discrimination across the ideological divide: The role of value violations and abstract values in discrimination by liberals and conservatives. *Social Psychological and Personality Science, 4,* 658–667.

White, C. G. (2008). *Unsettled minds: Psychology and the American search for spiritual assurance, 1830–1940.* Berkeley: University of California Press.

Index

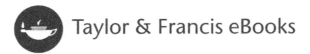

Taylor & Francis eBooks

Helping you to choose the right eBooks for your Library

Add Routledge titles to your library's digital collection today. Taylor and Francis ebooks contains over 50,000 titles in the Humanities, Social Sciences, Behavioural Sciences, Built Environment and Law.

Choose from a range of subject packages or create your own!

Benefits for you

» Free MARC records
» COUNTER-compliant usage statistics
» Flexible purchase and pricing options
» All titles DRM-free.

Benefits for your user

» Off-site, anytime access via Athens or referring URL
» Print or copy pages or chapters
» Full content search
» Bookmark, highlight and annotate text
» Access to thousands of pages of quality research at the click of a button.

REQUEST YOUR **FREE** INSTITUTIONAL TRIAL TODAY

Free Trials Available
We offer free trials to qualifying academic, corporate and government customers.

eCollections – Choose from over 30 subject eCollections, including:

Archaeology	Language Learning
Architecture	Law
Asian Studies	Literature
Business & Management	Media & Communication
Classical Studies	Middle East Studies
Construction	Music
Creative & Media Arts	Philosophy
Criminology & Criminal Justice	Planning
Economics	Politics
Education	Psychology & Mental Health
Energy	Religion
Engineering	Security
English Language & Linguistics	Social Work
Environment & Sustainability	Sociology
Geography	Sport
Health Studies	Theatre & Performance
History	Tourism, Hospitality & Events

For more information, pricing enquiries or to order a free trial, please contact your local sales team:
www.tandfebooks.com/page/sales

Routledge
Taylor & Francis Group

The home of
Routledge books

www.tandfebooks.com